Questioning the Premedical Paradigm

Questioning the Premedical Paradigm

*Enhancing Diversity in the Medical Profession
a Century after the Flexner Report*

DONALD A. BARR, M.D., PH.D.
Associate Professor
Departments of Sociology and Pediatrics
Stanford University
Stanford, California

The Johns Hopkins University Press
Baltimore

The Johns Hopkins University Press
2715 North Charles Street
Baltimore, Maryland 21218-4363
www.press.jhu.edu

Library of Congress Cataloging-in-Publication Data
Barr, Donald A.
Questioning the premedical paradigm: enhancing diversity in the medical profession a century after the Flexner report / Donald A. Barr.
p. ; cm.
Includes bibliographical references and index.
ISBN-13: 978-0-8018-9416-9 (hardcover : alk. paper)
ISBN-10: 0-8018-9416-6 (hardcover : alk. paper)
1. Premedical education—United States. I. Title.
[DNLM: 1. Education, Premedical—United States. 2. Cultural Diversity—United States. 3. Physicians—United States. W 18 B268q 2010]
R838.B37-2010
610.71′173—dc22
2009020308

A catalog record for this book is available from the British Library.

Special discounts are available for bulk purchases of this book. For more information, please contact Special Sales at 410-516-6936 or specialsales@press.jhu.edu.

The Johns Hopkins University Press uses environmentally friendly book materials, including recycled text paper that is composed of at least 30 percent post-consumer waste, whenever possible. All of our book papers are acid-free, and our jackets and covers are printed on paper with recycled content.

For Isaac

CONTENTS

This book has grown from my experiences advising undergraduates at Stanford University over a period of fifteen years. In that time I have seen many fine, fully qualified students enter Stanford with the aspiration of becoming physicians and leave Stanford to enroll in medical school as the fulfillment of that aspiration. However, I have also seen similar numbers of students, most of whom also appear fully qualified, enter as premedical students only to drop medicine as a possible career. I felt both a personal and a professional need to find out why some students stayed in premedical studies and others left. The research I initiated to explore this issue was the genesis of this book.

In chapter 1 I describe the results of research I conducted over a period of five years, following students entering either Stanford or the University of California, Berkeley, with a self-identified interest in becoming a physician. The results confirm my initial impression and raise an important issue. Courses in chemistry, biology, and physics, the same triad that seemed to define the "purpose of life" for premedical students when I was in college more than forty years ago, apparently serve that same function today. Where did this come from? What were the historical origins of this belief in the predictive value of success in chemistry, biology, and physics? I address this question in chapters 2 and 3.

In chapter 2 I trace the historical roots of premedical education from the late 1800s through 1905, the year our current model of premedical education was explicitly defined by the recently established Council on Medical Education (CME) as the norm by which medical schools should be judged. Following that action by the CME, a principal goal of medical educators was to ensure that students entering medical school had an adequate grounding in the fundamental principles of chemistry, biology, and physics. As we will see, the growing focus on premedical success in these subjects was based on a combination of political necessity and commonly held belief, with little in the way of scientific evidence linking premedical success with clinical success. Chapter 3 extends this analysis by following the historical evolution of premedical education from 1905 onward, through the reports from the 1920s of the need to avoid "wastage" (i.e., academic failure in the first year of medical school) among medical students, to a 1953 report that explicitly identified the necessity of "weeding out" less-qualified premedical students early in their college careers.

To what extent does success in the premedical sciences actually predict success in medical school and success as a clinical practitioner? I address this question in chapter 4, reviewing several decades of studies linking metrics of success in the premedical sciences with success in medical school and success in clinical practice. What we will find is that modeling the cause/effect associations between premedical success and success in and after medical school is complex. Some of the associations are as might be expected; some are unexpected. The message we will derive from these studies is that like begets like. Success in the premedical sciences gives rise to success in the preclinical sciences encountered early in medical school. However, the data repeatedly demonstrate that success in the premedical sciences has little predictive value regarding eventual success as a clinician. A substantial shift occurs midway in the medical school experience, from a focus on acquiring scientific knowledge to a focus on acquiring clinical knowledge and learning how to apply that knowledge in an actual clinical context. After this shift takes place, the role of success in the premedical sciences diminishes as a predictor of success in medical school.

If scientific knowledge is linked only loosely with clinical skills, are there other factors that might accurately predict clinical success? As described in chapter 5, this is a question medical educators have been struggling with for more than fifty years. There is an extensive series of studies on the psychological, or "noncognitive" aspects of premedical preparation and medical practice that parallels the studies described in the previous chapter focusing on the scientific, or "cognitive" aspects of premedical preparation in the sciences. From the period preceding the Flexner Report of 1910 to the present, medical educators have approached the practice of medicine as part science and part art. If success in the premedical sciences predicts success in the *science* of medicine, what (if anything) predicts success in the *art* of medicine? As we shall see, the answer to this question has proved to be elusive.

In his 1910 report, Abraham Flexner was concerned with the scientific basis of medical education and medical practice. He had little to say about the racial or ethnic diversity of the medical profession. Today the issue of diversity within the medical profession is central to medical education. A series of reports from organizations such as the Institute of Medicine of the National Academy of Sciences, the Association of American Medical Colleges, and the Office of the President of the University of California have underscored the urgency of increasing the racial and ethnic diversity of the medical profession as a national policy priority. In chapter 6 I review efforts from the 1960s onward to bring more students from underrepresented racial and ethnic minority (URM) groups into the premedical "pipeline" and help them prepare for medical school and a career as a physician.

Will adopting programs that make medical education more available to URM students necessarily imply a lowering of standards for entry into the medical profession? Chapter 6 goes on to review a series of studies that address this question. The data will confirm what we have discovered at Stanford: URM students often have a more difficult experience in the premedical sciences. However, more than two decades of research in the academic and career trajectories of students who enter medical school through programs of affirmative action or other programs designed to increase URM participation in medical education show conclusively that little if anything is sacrificed by making medical education more available to these students. In a landmark study from the University of California, Davis, students admitted under the system of racial and ethnic preferences that were eventually outlawed by the Supreme Court's *Bakke* decision demonstrated markers of professional success that were largely indistinguishable from their classmates who gained admission through the classical premedical curriculum.

While Flexner's model of premedical education continues to be the norm nationally, a number of medical schools have adopted alternative approaches to admissions. I review some of these in chapter 7. In particular, the medical school at McMaster University in Canada, has made admissions available both to students who are prepared in the premedical sciences and those who are not. Mount Sinai School of Medicine in New York has had a program for several years that identifies students at other universities after their sophomore year and accepts them based on their early academic performance and evidence of other personal strengths. Interestingly, students accepted into this program must commit to having an undergraduate major that is *not* in the natural sciences. While students accepted to these programs sometimes experience difficulty in the preclinical sciences early in medical school, the level of their eventual clinical skills is indistinguishable from those students whose undergraduate careers focused more on the sciences.

An overarching question I address in chapter 8 pertains to the title of this book: Is it accurate to describe the model of premedical education that was identified in 1905 by the CME and was codified in 1910 in the Flexner Report as a scientific paradigm? Ever since Thomas Kuhn published his seminal work *The Structure of Scientific Revolutions* in 1962, scientists and philosophers alike have been debating what actually constitutes a scientific paradigm. Kuhn describes a paradigm as "the entire constellation of beliefs, values, techniques, and so on shared by the members of a given community." Kuhn attributes two distinct aspects to a scientific paradigm. It is both a statement of a common understanding among scientists of "what the world is like," and a set of specific models of behavior that create "a new and more rigid definition of the field."[1]

Does the system of premedical education, and that of medical school admissions that follows from it, represent a paradigm as conceptualized by Kuhn? After reviewing the history of premedical education and the cumulative data linking premedical performance to performance in medical school, in chapter 8 I consider this question and its implications for medical education in the twenty-first century.

In chapter 9 I conclude this discussion by suggesting an alternative curricular and pedagogical approach to premedical education. In doing so, I will certainly not be proposing a "scientific revolution" in which one way of seeing the world replaces another. Rather, I will suggest that it would be more appropriate to offer parallel tracks of premedical education: one that emphasizes education in the natural sciences in the manner Flexner suggested in 1910, and a second one that instead approaches the acquisition of premedical knowledge through the integration of the human life sciences. I will suggest that the classical means of approaching the premedical sciences, with chemistry as a distinct and separate discipline from biology, and both as distinct from physics, with each taught in different buildings by different professors in different academic departments, may be neither appropriate nor optimal for many students.

If a student is learning the structure of the DNA molecule and how it translates genetic information into physiological processes through transcription and protein synthesis, is the student studying chemistry or studying biology? I will suggest that these disciplinary boundaries make little sense in many contexts. By approaching as an integrated whole the fundamental principles of scientific knowledge that are requisite for delving more deeply into the sciences underlying medical care, we may be able to provide many premedical students with a comprehensive scientific education in a manner that is substantially more efficient than the original model supported by Flexner.

I thank my colleagues who have read various parts of this book as it evolved. Their suggestions and advice were invaluable. Thanks go to Gert Brieger, Jules Dienstag, Elisabeth Hansot, Philip Lee, Anne MacLachlan, Charles Terrell, David Tyack, and Abigail Zuger. I also wish to express my appreciation for the input and support I have received from Professors John Matsui and Caroline Kanes of the University of California, Berkeley. Thanks also to Wendy Harris, my always-supportive editor at the Johns Hopkins University Press, and to Debra Satz, my always-supportive wife and intellectual partner.

Questioning the Premedical Paradigm

Introduction

I first began advising undergraduate students at Stanford in the fall of 1994. Early in my teaching career, one of the first of these students came to my office to ask me to be her faculty adviser. As one of the most popular majors at Stanford, the Human Biology program asks students to submit a written proposal describing the classes they will take and then to present that proposal to the faculty member they would like to work with as their adviser. This student had completed the initial prerequisites and proposed a series of classes focusing on issues surrounding the health care system. As she handed her proposal to me to review, she added a qualifier. "I'd like you to be my adviser, but only if you won't try to talk me into going to medical school."

Her admonition both puzzled and intrigued me. I was relatively new to undergraduate advising. I had interrupted my career as a practicing physician to return for graduate study in health policy and sociology. After completing my Ph.D., I applied and was selected for a faculty position at one of the leading public health schools in the country and was asked to develop a program of research and teaching for both medical students and graduate students in public health. The same week that I received written confirmation of the faculty position, I also received a court order informing me that if I accepted the offered position (thus moving out of state), I would be required to relinquish custody of my 13-year-old son. I declined the job offer, deciding instead to return to the practice of medicine and abandon my aspirations for an academic career.

A month or so later, I learned that the undergraduate Program in Human Biology at Stanford needed someone to teach a course about the health care system. Having organized just such a course intended for medical students, I agreed to offer it to Human Biology students instead. The course was listed too late to appear in the printed course catalogue, so I was told not to expect more than 25 or 30 students. Instead, I got 80 students, one of whom was now asking me to be her adviser. Feeling no personal stake in the student's career trajectory, I readily agreed to her request, reviewing and signing her forms. After handing them back to her, I asked out of curiosity, "Why did you want me not to try and talk you into going to medical school?"

"I used to be premed," she explained, "but then I got into the chemistry class-room, and I couldn't stand being around all those other premeds. They're much too competitive. I'm more of a fuzzy."

To understand her explanation one needs to appreciate the "techy/fuzzy" di-chotomy many students at Stanford have come to live by. As I understand it, a "techy" is someone who excels at math, science, or engineering. He or she is focused, driven, and competitive, perhaps also lacking in certain social sensibilities. A "fuzzy" on the other hand is a "people person," —someone who prefers studying the hu-manities or social sciences, someone who sees the world in broad contextual terms. While I easily recognize these stereotypic characteristics, I suspect "techy/fuzzy" is more accurately seen as a continuum. We all contain a certain amount of "techy-ness" and of "fuzzy-ness." For the sake of discussion, however, I accepted her di-chotomy.

"Let me see if I understand what you're saying," I asked. "Suppose you or some-one close to you had a brain aneurysm, and if the neurosurgeon didn't operate *just right,* you could end up with permanent brain damage. Would you rather have a techy neurosurgeon or a fuzzy neurosurgeon?"

"I'd rather have a techy neurosurgeon," she readily replied.

"Me too. But suppose instead someone close to you had a chronic illness for which there was no cure, and over a period of years the illness would lead to pro-gressive weakness and eventually to the person's death. Would you rather have a techy doctor or a fuzzy doctor working with this person?"

Again she readily replied, "I'd rather have a fuzzy doctor."

"So would I," I mused, "but if all the fuzzies drop out of premed, where are all the fuzzy doctors going to come from?"

I certainly had not intended to be flip. I had come to appreciate the profound change that health care in America was beginning to experience. Following the sci-entific revolution in medical education and medical practice that had taken place at its opening, the twentieth century had seen tremendous advances in medical science and medical care technology. The twenty-first century, on the other hand, would be a century of learning to cope with chronic illness for which there typically would be no cure and having to do so under the increasing pressure of constrained economic resources. From my two decades of medical practice I knew that well-trained, com-mitted, and compassionate doctors—fuzzies—were what would be needed in the coming decades of American health care.

Here was a self-described fuzzy whom I intuitively sensed could make a superb physician. The irony was that the hypercompetitive atmosphere of the freshman chemistry classroom had resulted in this student's losing interest in a career as a physician. This despite the fact that she was no stranger to competition—she was a world-class athlete, already in possession of multiple Olympic medals. She could cope with the competition of athletics; what she couldn't cope with was the competition of premedical studies, what has often been referred to as the "premedical syndrome."[1]

Those who have followed the story of Harry Potter are familiar with the "sorting hat." Those who have not will need to know that this magical hat is used at the Hogwarts School of Witchcraft and Wizardry to assign first-year students to a specific residential house, and in so doing also assigning them to a specific career trajectory as a wizard or a witch. A young student stands in front of the assembled students and faculty and places the hat over his or her head. With its magical powers the hat is able to sense the student's true nature, and based on that nature announces its decision. For Harry, the hat (fortunately) announced "Gryffindor!" For Draco Malfoy, it announced "Slytherin." And thus the die was cast.

For the student sitting across from me, it was as if her freshman class in introductory chemistry had acted as a sorting hat. Entering the classroom and looking around her, she had slipped the hat over her head. For some of her fellow students the hat announced, "Premed!" For her, the hat had instead whispered in her ear, "You're not premed." She was more of a fuzzy and thus would not be going to medical school.

That was the last conversation she and I had about medical school. I kept in touch with her over the following years and learned, somewhat to my surprise, that after graduating from Stanford she had re-thought her decision and decided to go to medical school after all. To complete her required premedical classes she had enrolled in a well-known women's college that has a program targeted at women such as her—a program that not only welcomed but sought out fuzzies who wanted to become physicians. She did superbly in her science prerequisites and was easily accepted into one of the top medical schools in the country. She is now a physician.

Over time, my teaching in Human Biology became more and more successful, the classes I offered more and more popular. It wasn't long before I had hundreds of students taking my classes and scores of students coming to my office hours, asking me to be their faculty adviser. With each of these advisees, after reviewing and approving their proposal for their Human Biology major, I took a moment to ask what his or her career plans were. A striking pattern emerged. While many of the students said, "I'm premed; I plan to go to medical school," just as many said, "I used to be premed, but . . ." Each would fill in the space after the "but . . ." with a slightly different story, but each said essentially the same thing. As an incoming freshman, they had had aspirations of becoming a physician. Now, however, after weathering the first year or two of premedical sciences, they had abandoned that aspiration and were instead looking at a different career trajectory. They each had put on the premed sorting hat and had heard "You're not premed." Now, nearly halfway through their college experience, each was coming to me for career advice.

I began to notice within this overall pattern of diverging career trajectories a second, more disturbing pattern. It seemed that nearly all the students who explained, "I used to be premed, but . . ." were women, and many of these were from underrepresented racial or ethnic groups. The premedical sorting hat appeared to be giving a different message to women, especially women of color, than it did to men and students not in an underrepresented minority (URM) group. Despite a growing national urgency to increase the diversity of the medical profession by encouraging more URM students to go to medical school, substantial numbers of highly talented URM students coming to my office had heard from the sorting hat that medicine was not for them.

I began to take more of an interest in what these students did after graduating from Stanford. Several anecdotal descriptions illustrate my growing sense of discomfort with the way early experiences in the science classroom at Stanford appeared to direct otherwise highly talented students away from a career in medicine. These students are typical of the many students with whom I have had the privilege of working.

The first student was Latina, one of the first in her family to pursue higher education. She had experienced a very difficult first two years in the science classroom at Stanford, earning mostly grades of C+ and B−. (Her grades in her non-science classes were considerably higher.) Despite her early difficulties in her science classes, she had not given up the intention of becoming a physician and had applied to a range of medical schools. Each school had rejected her, presumably based on her low grades in the premedical sciences. After she graduated, I hired her to work on a project I had developed to expand opportunities for undergraduates to complete an internship working with a community-based medical clinic that provided care to mostly low-income and uninsured patients. Based largely on her efforts in establishing working relationships with these clinics, the program grew to be a substantial success. Sensing her undiminished commitment to a medical career, I encouraged her to apply for a program at the University of California offering post-baccalaureate premedical education to URM students who had unsuccessfully applied to medical school. She was readily accepted to the "post-bac" program and experienced substantial academic success. When she applied to medical school a second time, she was accepted to a program at a top national medical school that offered students training in both medicine and public health. She was elected president of her freshman medical school class, completed her professional education, and is now a successful physician. In her case, the sorting hat got it wrong.

The next two students came to my office a year or so later. Each was female, each was African American. Each had entered Stanford as premed but had experienced substantial difficulty in the science classroom (mostly in chemistry), earning a series of C's and B's, some gained only after repeating a class. Each decided to apply to graduate school in public health rather than medical school.

The first student had worked with me for two years on an undergraduate research project of her own design. Using a large statewide database, she had shown that African American patients in California were less likely to be offered a potentially life-saving therapy than white patients with the same disease and same insurance. She graduated from Stanford with academic honors and attended a top school of public health. She did as well with her graduate studies as she had done in her coursework and research with me. Her advisers in public health urged her to ignore the message of the sorting hat and to apply to medical school after earning her graduate degree. She was accepted into a top medical school, receiving a highly competitive scholarship.

The second student had chosen to spend three months of her undergraduate career in a special program Stanford offers in Washington, D.C. As part of this program she completed a 10-week internship in the Office of Minority Health in the U.S. Department of Health and Human Services, participating in a project examining the sources of health disparities among African Americans in the United States. I received glowing evaluations from her internship supervisor. Like her colleague before her, she applied to the same school of public health. Despite her relatively low grades in chemistry at Stanford, she completed her graduate studies with a grade point average of 4.07, earning straight A's, except for three grades of A+. She applied to fourteen medical schools and was accepted at all fourteen. I guess the sorting hat was wrong again.

The last student, also an African American female, entered Stanford with the hope of becoming a physician but experienced difficulty in her early science classes, principally in chemistry. She became my advisee as a junior, showing a keen interest in and talent for issues of health care policy and health inequality. Rather than attending medical school, she chose to focus her career on advocating for better health care and improved health status for disadvantaged patients. She was accepted jointly to the Harvard Law School and the Harvard School of Public Health, enrolling in a joint J.D.-M.P.H. program, and will undoubtedly be a successful health advocate. While I have no doubt that she could have succeeded in becoming a physician had she wanted to, I fully support her decision to take a different tack.

The more students I talked with, the more I learned about what it was like to be premed at Stanford. As an undergraduate at Oberlin College, I had largely escaped the culture of premed, deciding relatively late in my college career to attend medical school. Initially, I wanted to be a professor of mathematics, having earned straight A's in an accelerated high school math program. After my freshman year of college, however, I had relinquished my aspirations toward a career in math: *I got a C+ in freshman calculus.* Not knowing that I could easily have overcome that dark stain (I got a B+ in second-year math), I assumed that a career in math was not for me.

My college adviser sat me down at the end of my sophomore year and asked, "Well, if you're not going to be a math major, what's your major going to be?" I had done well in my science courses, earning high grades in chemistry. I was enjoying my current biology course much more than I had enjoyed my freshman chemistry, so I replied, "I guess I'll be a biology major," to which he replied, "Straight biology or premed biology?" There it was, the sorting hat, although I did not recognize it. (It would be three decades before J. K. Rowling would name it.)

I hesitated, then rather impulsively replied, "Premed." The die was cast. I went to medical school, became a successful physician, and somehow gravitated back to academics. Despite having initially assumed that by turning down the proffered faculty position I was walking away from an academic career, the popularity of my teaching and my advising grew continuously. Before I knew it, I was a full-time academic and only a part-time physician, with dozens of premed and formerly premed advisees.

Stanford University asks all of its incoming freshmen the following question: "If you are considering a career after you complete Stanford, what is that career?" Each year between 350 and 400 of the 1,600 or so incoming freshmen answer that question by stating that they hope to become physicians. Based on their answers, Stanford's undergraduate advising system assigns each of these students a special "premed adviser"—an adviser specifically versed in premedical requirements and the process of preparing for medical school. Even though the university specifically disavows having a specific premedical major, each of these incoming students receives the preliminary label as premed.

It is not the university's preliminary labeling that carries the most force, however. Somehow the new students rapidly come to know that, if you are premed at Stanford, you have to take chemistry your freshman year, followed by biology your sophomore year, and also fitting in a year of physics somewhere along the way. Student after student has explained to me, unprompted, that they felt it was nearly compulsory to take the first course in the undergraduate chemistry sequence during their first academic quarter at Stanford. To wait and start your chemistry in the second quarter of your freshman year meant that you were already "off-track." It seemed almost as if their very existence as a premedical student depended on following this pre-set path, starting at the chemistry classroom.

Several years after I started teaching in Human Biology I had occasion to read *Arrowsmith*, Sinclair Lewis's Nobel Prize–winning novel about Martin Arrowsmith, a young college student at the University of Winnemac, a fictional Midwestern university. As Lewis describes it, "In 1904, Martin Arrowsmith was an Arts and Sciences Junior preparing for medical school. . . . Martin's father and mother were dead, leaving him only enough money for his arts and medical courses. The purpose of life was chemistry and physics and the prospect of biology next year."[2]

Lewis wrote these words in 1924. As we will see, his description of the premedical experience more accurately reflects the period of the 1920s, for in 1904, few medical schools expected students to have a college degree before entering. One of the few Midwestern universities to have both a rigorous premedical curriculum and an affiliated school of medicine was the University of Michigan. However, in 1904 Michigan did not require courses in chemistry, physics, and biology as prerequisites to matriculation to medical school.

Two momentous reports were issued in the interval between Martin's fictional experience in 1904 and Lewis's describing it in 1924. The first was the publication of the Flexner Report, authored by Abraham Flexner and published in 1910 by the Carnegie Foundation for the Advancement of Teaching. In the report, Flexner issued a scathing indictment of the state of medical education in the United States, using the model of medical education in Europe as his standard for comparison. Flexner urged adoption of laws mandating that medical schools be part of larger universities and offer a four-year curriculum rather than the traditional two-year curriculum. Of these four years of medical school, the first two must be devoted to the study of science. To prepare for this new and more rigorous type of medical education, Flexner also suggested that the only proper undergraduate preparation for medical school is an equally rigorous undergraduate course in the sciences: "The normal rhythm of physiologic function must remain a riddle to students who cannot think and speak in biological, chemical, and physical language."[3]

In 1914, the American Medical Association's Council on Medical Education, originally founded in 1905, issued a major report on the occasion of its tenth anniversary. This report called on all medical schools to adopt Flexner's recommendations regarding university affiliation, curriculum, and premedical preparation, specifically identifying two years of chemistry, one year of physics, and one year of biology as the minimum college preparation adequate for entering medical school. (The report also mandated a reading knowledge of French and German.) By the time Lewis wrote *Arrowsmith*, more than 85 percent of medical schools in the

United States had adopted Flexner's model of premedical education, with most mandating a minimum of two years of college while preferring four years and a bachelor's degree. In 1924, the "purpose of life" for most American premedical students had become "chemistry and physics, and the prospect of biology next year."

By the 1950s this expectation had become a deeply held cultural norm among premedical students as well as colleges and universities. The surge in the number of students entering college in the decades after World War II began to put a severe strain on the medical school application process. There were between two and three times as many college students hoping to become physicians as there were available slots in medical schools. For most of these premedical students, the "purpose of life" had become excelling in the required courses in chemistry, physics, and biology, and by so doing securing a coveted place in the entering class of a medical school. If more than half of the aspiring premedical students would fail in their effort to enter medical school, success in the premedical sciences described in 1910 by Flexner was crucial. A less-than-stellar performance in the triad of premedical sciences would likely result in failure to gain admission to medical school. Premedical studies had become a pressure cooker. Reports of the behavioral and psychological price students paid to enter premed described a "premedical syndrome." In 1955, Funkenstein described the pressures premedical students at Harvard faced: "Seeking council from his colleagues, premedical advisers, doctors and friends, he becomes more and more anxiety ridden as he contemplates the almost super-human test before him of securing entrance to medical school. With great trepidation he . . . enters what the Harvard Crimson calls the 'rat race.'"[4]

For premedical students entering Stanford in the 1990s, the pressure of premedical expectations seemed just as severe as that experienced by young Martin Arrowsmith earlier in the century and by Harvard students in the 1950s. If you wanted to become a physician, it was common knowledge that you had to begin chemistry during your first semester or quarter of college and that you must do well. After mastering chemistry, the next hurdles were biology and physics. Failure to attain early success in these subjects meant failure as a premedical student. As described in 1953 by Aura Severinghaus of Columbia University, a college or university was doing its job by "weeding out" those students not fit to study medicine.[5]

In making his recommendation in 1910 that "the normal rhythm of physiologic function must remain a riddle to students who cannot think and speak in biological, chemical, and physical language," Flexner asks us to take this association on faith. Without offering any scientific support for his assertion, he asks us to believe that a lack of success in the premedical sciences implies lack of future success in medical school and as a physician. Similarly, he seems to suggest that success in the premedical sciences logically implies success in medical school and as a physician.

These relationships seem intuitive. It seems to make sense that to succeed in medicine one must first succeed in the premedical sciences. However, can we take it on faith that these relationships are accurate—that they are supported by scientific evidence?

During the period from 1920 to 1940, it was typical for 25 percent or more of entering medical students to be dismissed from medical school after the first year due to academic failure. It seemed that one way to decrease the likelihood of academic failure in medical school was to select only those students who had demonstrated success in the premedical sciences. Using success in these sciences as a predictor of future success in the early years medical school, many colleges and universities adopted the explicit goal of "weeding out" students who were weak in the sciences, especially chemistry. As described in 1953 in a major national report, "Some chemistry teachers claim with pride that only students of good ability who work very hard can get through their chemistry course."[6] From reports of students' personal experiences, this certainly seems still to be the case at Stanford. Many of my advisees have described hearing their chemistry professor explicitly state that those who could not succeed in chemistry should drop their goal of attending medical school.

If it were true that lack of success in chemistry were consistently linked with lack of success in medical school, it would be difficult to argue with the logic of this screening process, whether it is applied explicitly or implicitly. The same is true of undergraduate success in biology. If it were true that difficulty in biology is consistently associated with difficulty passing courses in medical school, it would be reasonable to discourage those students who experience early difficulty in science courses from continuing to pursue premedical studies. But are these associations accurate?

The clear success of the URM students described above, each of whom experienced early difficulty in chemistry or other premedical sciences, calls into question the association between success in premedical sciences and success as a physician. Each of those who chose to go to medical school has been successful, and each will, I am confident, be a superb physician. Might it be that Flexner was wrong?

We will see in chapter 4 that there is ample evidence that academic success or demonstrated knowledge in the premedical sciences is strongly associated with success in the preclinical sciences. We will also see, however, that Flexner's second assumption—that a relative lack of success in the premedical sciences implies that a student will not be able to succeed in medical school and as a physician—is not supported by scientific data. While students who perform less well in the premedical sciences than their classmates do have an increased chance of experiencing difficulty in the preclinical phase of medical school, the vast majority (as many as 98%) will succeed in their preclinical studies. Furthermore, the data will show that success in the preclinical sciences encountered early in medical school has little relationship to eventual success as a clinician. In study after study, students who enter medical school despite a relatively weak background in the premedical sciences enjoy success as clinicians that is comparable to their more scientifically inclined classmates.

If the premedical experience is only a weak predictor of success as a clinician, why do we continue to use the premedical sciences as the "sorting hat" for medical school? What are the historical origins of the widely held belief that chemistry, biology, and physics are the necessary precursors of a successful medical school experience? This is one of the principal questions I address in this book.

However, before attempting to answer this question I must first be sure that the impressions I have gained through my years of teaching and advising Human Biology students at Stanford are supported by data. Is it true that the premedical sciences, in particular chemistry, have the effect of "weeding out" many women and URM students who otherwise possess academic strengths and personal characteristics that are well suited to a career as a physician? In the following chapter I present data from my study of premedical students at Stanford University and at the University of California, Berkeley. As we will see, the sorting hat is alive and well at both universities. For better or for worse, early experiences in the chemistry classroom continue to have a disproportionate impact on students' decision of whether to remain in premedical studies or to drop their aspirations for a medical career. Isn't it time we tried a different way to select and train students for medicine?

Mine is not the only voice asking these types of questions. There is a growing sense among many medical and premedical educators that the model of premedical education defined in 1905 by the CME and promulgated in 1910 by Flexner—the *premedical paradigm*—may be overdue for a major shift. Whether that shift is evolutionary or revolutionary remains to be determined. I hope the analyses and discussions contained in this book will contribute to this process.

CHAPTER ONE

Who Drops Out of Premed, and Why?

In the introduction I described my experiences advising undergraduate students in the Human Biology program of Stanford University. For many of these students, something happens early in their undergraduate experience that causes them to turn away from medicine as a career. From repeated anecdotes, I have learned that a student's early experience in chemistry courses is often a factor in that decision. However, these are simply anecdotes. Do they accurately reflect a larger pattern? Is it true that the premedical sciences, in particular chemistry, have the effect of "weeding out" many women and students from underrepresented minority (URM) groups who otherwise possess academic strengths and personal characteristics that seem well suited to a career as a physician? Before I could think about what approach to take in addressing this issue, I needed to know if these anecdotal impressions were accurate and could be supported by data. I needed to undertake a carefully thought out program of research addressing the question of who loses interest in premedical studies and why. If I were able to confirm that this "weeding out" process affects URM students disproportionately, these results would have potential significance for the ongoing policy debate about how best to increase the racial and ethnic diversity of the medical profession both in California and in the United States more generally.

The Need to Increase the Diversity of the Medical Profession

Increasing the racial and ethnic diversity of the medical profession in the United States has become a pressing national policy priority. In 1996 Jordan Cohen, then

Material in this chapter was previously published as D. A. Barr, M. Gonzalez, and S. F. Wanat, "The Leaky Pipeline: Factors Associated with Early Decline in Interest in Pre-medical Studies among Under-Represented Minority Undergraduate Students," in *Academic Medicine* 83 (2008): 503–11, and reproduced with permission of the publisher; and D. A. Barr, J. Matsui, M. Gonzalez, and S. F. Wanat, "Chemistry Courses as the Turning Point for Premedical Students," in Advances in Health Sciences Education, published electronically in advance of print and reproduced here with permission of the publisher.

president of the Association of American Medical Colleges, called on the AAMC and on the leaders of U.S. medical schools "to bridge the appalling diversity gap that still separates medicine from the society it professes to serve."[1] Nearly a decade later, the AAMC issued a follow-up report that re-emphasized, both to the admissions committees of medical schools and to the country as a whole, the continuing imperative of expanding the racial and ethnic diversity of the medical profession: "As our nation becomes increasingly diverse, the need for and potential impact of a diverse physician workforce will become more pronounced. . . . [A]nticipating the change in the nation's demographics represents an additional imperative for medical education to educate more minority physicians and physicians that are culturally sensitive and focused on patient care."[2]

Twice in recent years the Institute of Medicine of the National Academy of Sciences has issued scientific reports stressing the importance of this issue. The editors of a 2001 study stated, "Many minority groups, including African Americans, Hispanics, and Native Americans, are poorly represented in the health professions relative to their proportions in the overall U.S. population. . . . Increasing the diversity of health professionals has been an explicit strategy of the federal government and many private groups."[3] A 2004 report titled *In the Nation's Compelling Interest* concluded that "a preponderance of scientific evidence supports the importance of increasing racial and ethnic diversity among health professionals."[4]

Despite this need for increased racial/ethnic diversity, the number of physicians from URM groups graduating from U.S. medical schools, including African American, Latino, and Native American graduates, has shown a steady decline from the peak rates seen in the mid-1990s. Paralleling the decline in the number of URM graduates from medical school has been a decline in the number of URM applicants to medical school.[5]

The decline in applicants and graduates has been even more acute in California. With a population that is both growing and aging, and with an increasing prevalence of chronic diseases, the State of California is expected to have a shortage of up to 17,000 physicians by the year 2015.[6] Compounding this problem is the concurrent need to increase the racial and ethnic diversity of the medical profession in California. Of the projected increase of 12 million people in the state's population in the next 25 years, 75 percent is expected to be among Latinos.[7] Grumbach and colleagues, in analyzing the results of a survey of more than 60,000 California physicians, concluded that "the underrepresentation of Latinos and African Americans among California physicians remains dire."[8] Among Grumbach's recommendations to address these issues is "invest[ing] in the educational pipeline preparing minority and disadvantaged students for careers in medicine and other health professions."[9] However, my experience at Stanford suggested that the "pipeline" of minority and disadvantaged students in California who are heading toward a career in medicine had sprung a leak. From anecdotal evidence conveyed to me by colleagues at the University of California (UC), I had every reason to believe that UC's "pipeline" had also sprung a leak, with a profound impact on the ability of UC medical schools to train a diverse physician workforce.

In the early 1990s, UC's five medical schools were enjoying substantial success in enrolling qualified medical students from URM groups, with 117 URM first-year students enrolling at a UC school. However, in the wake of new policies adopted by the UC regents and of Proposition 209 approved by California voters, the number of first-year URM students enrolling in UC medical schools fell to 63 in 2000.[10] While that number has increased somewhat to an average of about 100 students per year for the past several years, this level remains well below the levels realized before Proposition 209. This drop in URM enrollment at UC medical schools was accompanied by a parallel drop in URM students from California who applied to medical school. In 1994, 711 URM students from California applied to medical school somewhere in the country; in 1999, this number had fallen to 476, a decrease of 33 percent. URM premedical students at Stanford appeared to be losing interest in a medical career early in their undergraduate experience. Was the same thing happening to students at UC Berkeley, the flagship campus of the UC system?

Understanding Why Students Leave Premedical Studies

Every year, Stanford University administers a survey to all incoming freshmen that addresses students' academic and professional aspirations, asking: "At this point in your life, if you are thinking of pursuing a graduate degree, in which area(s) would you do so?" In 2001, 313 incoming freshmen indicated an interest in attending medical school after Stanford. Of these, 93, or 30 percent, were URM students (i.e., those who self-identify as African American, Latino, or Native American). That same year, 280 students who had done their undergraduate education at Stanford applied to medical school through the AAMC's American Medical College Admissions Service. Of these 280 applicants, 38 were URM students, comprising slightly less than 14 percent of applicants.[11] Notably, while there were 220 incoming premedical students who were not in a URM group, there were 242 applicants who were not in a URM group. In other words, in 2001 the decrement in students applying to medical school from students entering as premedical students was fully accounted for by the loss of URM students from the premedical pipeline that runs through the four years of the Stanford undergraduate experience.

TABLE I.I.

Comparing the racial/ethnic and gender composition of entering premedical students at Stanford University (2001–2005) with that of medical school applicants from Stanford University (2001–2008)

	No.	Proportion of Total (%)	Change from No. of Freshman Premedical Students to No. of Medical School Applicants	Change as Proportion of Freshman Premedical Students (%)
Entering premedical students (N = 363.2)				
URM	108.2	29.8		
Female	67.6	62.5		
Male	40.6	37.5		
Non-URM	255.0	70.2		
Female	143.8	56.4		
Male	111.2	43.6		
Medical school applicants (N = 294.4)				
URM	50.1	17.0	58.1	53.7
Female	29.6	59.1	−38.0	−56.2
Male	20.5	40.9	−20.1	−49.5
Non-URM	244.3	83.0	10.7	4.2
Female	134.9	55.2	−8.9	−6.2
Male	109.4	44.8	−1.8	−1.6

Source: Premedical data provided by Stanford University. Medical school applicant data provided by the Association of American Medical Colleges.
Note: Numbers are averages for the periods shown.

Of course, it is difficult to generalize from a comparison of a single cohort of incoming freshmen premedical students with a single cohort of exiting medical school applicants. However, the discrepancy at that time was enough for me to begin to seek an explanation. Before I could fully document that URM students who enter Stanford are more prone to losing interest in a medical career than non-URM students, I would need to follow additional cohorts of incoming and exiting students. Accordingly, I gathered data from the fall of 2001 through the fall of 2005 on all students entering Stanford as freshmen and indicating an interest in a medical career, broken down by racial and ethnic group. In addition, I obtained data from the AAMC on all students from Stanford who applied to a U.S. medical school from the 2001 application cycle through the 2008 application cycle. I calculated the average number of incoming premedical students over this five-year period and compared it with the average number of medical school applicants over this eight-year period. The results are shown in table I.I.

It can be seen that the results from 2001 were not anomalous. Between 2001 and

2005, an average of 108 URM students entered Stanford each year hoping to become physicians. Between 2001 and 2008, an average of 50 URM students from Stanford applied to medical school—58 fewer than entered Stanford with premedical aspirations, representing a decrease of 54 percent. URM students, on average, make up 29.8 percent of the entering cohort of premedical students and 17.0 percent of the cohort of applicants. This decrease in the number of URM students applying to medical school is seen disproportionately among URM women. By comparison, every year about 11 fewer non-URM students apply to medical school than enter as premeds—a decrease of about 4 percent. As with URM students, this decline is seen principally among women.

On the assumption that, in choosing among some of most talented high school students in the country, the Stanford Undergraduate Admissions Office rarely misjudges a student's academic ability and potential, it appears that Stanford loses 58 otherwise qualified URM students from the premedical pipeline every year. While a substantial majority of these students stay at Stanford and graduate successfully, they appear to have given up their aspirations for a career as a physician.

Why does this happen? What makes these students change their minds? Do they find something more attractive that pulls them out of premed, or does something happen that pushes them out? Does anything like this also happen at UC Berkeley? These were the questions I felt compelled to answer.

Research Methodology Used to Study Premedical Students at Stanford

As noted above, Stanford University administers a survey to all incoming freshmen that records students' academic and professional aspirations. For this phase of the research, the university's Office of Institutional Research provided us with identifying information on all incoming students in the fall of 2002, 2003, and 2004 who responded to the question about career plans by indicating medicine as a probable area of study. This group of 1,101 students forms the initial study population. The Stanford Office of Human Subjects Research reviewed and approved our research protocol.

We developed a survey instrument that we administered to these students electronically. Approximately one week after freshman orientation, we sent an e-mail to each incoming student in the study population, asking him or her to participate in our study. Those who agreed to participate clicked on a Web link that took them to the consent page of our survey. We sent out two additional waves of e-mails to those students not responding to our initial request for participation.

After linking to the Web page with our survey and after giving consent for participation, students were asked to do the following: "Please choose a whole number between 1 and 10 from the Interest Scale which best describes your current interest in being premed." The students were then shown a 10-point scale, with the following prompts located at the numbers indicated:

10 So committed to premed that nothing can stop me

9

8

7 Probably will be premed

6

5

4 Probably will not be premed

3

2

1 Absolutely no interest whatsoever in premed

Students could indicate only a single whole number in response. In earlier piloting of our survey instrument, students consistently recognized that "being premed" meant to undertake a course of premedical studies in preparation for applying to medical school. The survey also asked students to indicate which, if any, immediate family members are doctors.

We maintained a list of those students who responded to our initial survey request. We sent each of these students an e-mail between two and four weeks from the end of the freshman year, asking them to link to our survey and to respond again to the question about their current level of interest in premedical studies, using the same 10-point visual scale. We sent two additional rounds of e-mails to those students who had responded to our initial survey at the beginning of the year but had not yet responded to our end-of-year survey. Finally, we repeated the survey at the end of the sophomore year, again sending out two additional rounds of e-mails to those subjects not responding. We report data on the 362 students who responded to all three surveys (overall response rate 34.3%).

We used a test-retest methodology to assess the reliability of our 10–point interest scale, requesting approximately 15 percent of the respondents in one admission cohort, identified randomly, to complete a duplicate survey three months after having completed the initial survey. Twenty-four of the thirty-eight repeat subjects completed the retest survey. The Pearson correlation coefficient between students' responses at these two times was 0.69 ($p < .001$).

In an initial pilot study of our survey instrument, we tested for possible response bias by telephoning 61 students who had not responded to the repeat survey administered at the end of freshman year. On the phone we asked them to rate the strength of their interest in premedical studies; we then compared their responses to 143 students who had responded and participated in the survey at the end of their freshman year. The mean interest level of the initial responders was 6.73 (95% CI: 6.36–7.11), while that of the nonresponders was 6.44 (95% CI: 5.77–7.12), suggesting that nonresponders to the follow-up surveys were less interested in continuing as premed than were those who did respond.

In addition to the data obtained from the student survey, the Office of Institutional Research provided us with the following data on each student: gender, principal racial or ethnic group (as identified by the student), zip code of family residence, SAT verbal score, and SAT math score. We categorized students into five principal racial/ethnic groups: white (not Hispanic), African American, Latino (Hispanic), Asian, Native American. We used the median household income for the zip code of the student's family residence to estimate the household income of the student's family. This estimation method has been shown to provide an appropriate estimate of family income when actual family-level data are not available.[12] We excluded students whose family lived outside the United States and students who indicated "other" for race/ethnicity, giving a final study population of 1,056 students.

We compared the mean interest level for each of the five racial/ethnic groups and for each of the three time periods studied. We refer to the interest level at the beginning of freshman year as Time 1 (T1), at the end of freshman year as Time 2 (T2), and at the end of sophomore year as Time 3 (T3). We calculated a measure of change in individual student interest by subtracting the response at T1 from the response at T3. A positive value indicated an increase in interest, while a negative value indicated a decline in interest.

Research Methodology Used to Study Premedical Students at Berkeley

In order to address the question of whether underrepresented minority students who enter UC Berkeley with an interest in pursuing premedical studies also experience a change in career interest, we approached colleagues at UC Berkeley and asked their help to gather comparable data on incoming Berkeley freshmen. If URM students at UC Berkeley were to experience the same leakage from the premedical "pipeline" as we found among those students at Stanford, the ability of the UC system to meet its goal of increasing the diversity of the California medical profession would be substantially impaired.

While we were able to conduct our research at Berkeley in a way that paralleled that at Stanford, we encountered some important methodological differences at Berkeley. While Stanford gathers information on future career plans from all incoming freshmen, UC Berkeley at that time did not. Accordingly, we were required to send an initial e-mail to every incoming Berkeley freshman, asking whether s/he was considering a career in medicine following graduation. Those students who were considering medicine were then asked to link to a Web site at which our survey was explained and at which approved informed consent for participation was obtained.

At Stanford, when a student responded to any of the surveys, the computer server housing the survey was able to record that student's unique identifier used for computer access. In this way we were able to link responses at the two time periods for individual students and compare changes over time at the level of the individual student. For Berkeley students, the computer server was not able to obtain a unique identifier for each survey respondent that would permit us reliably to link responses at the two times for individual students. Accordingly, in reporting our Berkeley data, we report mean responses of a specific racial or ethnic cohort and are able only to compare changes over time in cohort mean responses rather than individual student responses. We report data on students who entered Berkeley as freshmen in the fall of 2003, 2004, and 2005. Of these three cohorts, we were able to obtain data about the level of interest at the end of sophomore year in the first two cohorts.

Survey Results

Table 1.2 shows the average response to our survey for students at the beginning of the freshman year and the end of the sophomore year, sorted by racial/ethnic group and by school. A total of 1,036 Berkeley students responded to our survey at the beginning of their freshman year. Of these initial respondents, 589 also responded at the end of their sophomore year. We compare the interest level of these Berkeley students with that of the 362 Stanford students (out of an original sample of 1,056, overall response rate 34.3%) who responded to our survey at both times.

For African American, Latino, and Asian student groups, the initial level of interest is similar at the two universities. Native American respondents at Berkeley reported a lower initial level of interest than those at Stanford, while the white respondents at Berkeley reported a somewhat higher initial level of interest than those at Stanford.

Several interesting patterns can be seen in comparing the responses of Berkeley students and Stanford students. While Berkeley students and Stanford students generally start their freshman year with about the same level of interest, the decline

TABLE I.2.

Racial/ethnic differences in the level of interest in pursuing premedical studies for students at the University of California, Berkeley, and Stanford University

Racial or Ethnic Group	UC Berkeley			Stanford		
	Beginning of Freshman Year	End of Sophomore Year	Change in Level of Interest	Beginning of Freshman Year	End of Sophomore Year	Change in Level of Interest
White	7.02 (6.77–7.27) n=224	4.04 (3.54–4.53) n=166	−2.98	6.71 (6.43–7.00) n=142	5.66 (5.16–6.17) n=142	−1.05
Asian	7.07 (6.93–7.21) n=667	4.80 (4.48–5.12) n=340	−2.27	7.27 (7.00–7.55) n=136	6.90 (6.46–7.35) n=136	−0.37
African American	7.36 (6.68–7.49) n=36	6.00 (4.55–7.45) n=22	−1.36	7.25 (6.63–7.87) n=32	5.81 (4.82–6.81) n=32	−1.44
Latino	7.31 (6.94–7.69) n=102	5.00 (4.10–5.90) n=56	−2.31	7.49 (6.94–8.04) n=41	6.17 (5.11–7.24) n=41	−1.32
Native American	6.29 (4.04–8.53) n=7	3.20 (0.00–6.86) n=5	−3.09	8.09 (7.17–9.01) n=11	6.45 (4.24–8.67) n=11	−1.64

Note: Students were surveyed at the beginning of freshman year and at the end of sophomore year, using a 10-point scale of interest: 10 = highest level of interest; 1 = lowest level of interest. Data show mean response for each group (95% CI).

in that level of interest is quite a bit steeper at Berkeley. White (loss of 2.98 points), Asian (loss of 2.27 points), and Latino (loss of 2.31 points) students at Berkeley lose more interest than white (loss of 1.05 points), Asian (loss of 0.37 points), and Latino (loss of 1.32 points) students at Stanford.

By comparison, African American students at Berkeley (loss of 1.36 points) and at Stanford (loss of 1.44 points) have a similar level of decline. However, while African American students at Stanford have the second-largest decline among all racial/ethnic groups, at Berkeley they have the smallest decline and end their sophomore year with the greatest interest in continuing premedical studies of all the racial/ethnic groups.

Native American students at both Berkeley (loss of 3.09 points) and Stanford (loss of 1.64 points) report the largest decline of all the groups. Compared to the other racial/ethnic groups at Berkeley, Native American students start out with the lowest level of interest and remain in that position at the end of sophomore year. At

Stanford, Native American students start out with the highest level of interest and end with the second-highest level.

Analysis of Factors Associated with a Decline in Interest

Because we were able at Stanford to track responses over time for individual students and thus were able to link changes in interest level over time for each of these students, it was possible to test for those factors associated with the change over time in an individual student's level of interest. Accordingly, we first calculated the change in interest for each student between the beginning of the freshman year (T1) and the end of the sophomore year (T3) by subtracting the value at T1 from that at T3. A positive value for this variable indicates an increase in interest, and a negative value indicates a corresponding decrease. We found that the distribution of this variable approximated a normal distribution. We used ordinary least squares regression to evaluate the associations between the demographic variables we had for the students and the value of (T3–T1). The results of these analyses are shown in table 1.3.

In the first step of the analysis (model 1) we entered only a variable indicating underrepresented minority status, confirming that URM students at Stanford have a larger drop in interest between T1 and T3 than non-URM students. In model 2 we add a variable for female gender. In this analysis, both URM status and female gender are independently associated with a larger decline in interest. In a separate analysis, we tested for an interaction effect between URM status and female gender. We found no interaction; entering the interaction term weakened the fit of the model (data not shown).

In the third step (model 3) we entered median household income by zip code as a marker of family socioeconomic status (SES). While the coefficient for income was not significant, its inclusion resulted in the URM variable no longer having a significant association, suggesting an association between URM status and median household income. We tested for such an association and found that mean household income in zip codes of URM families was $62,439 (95% CI: $57,311–$67,577) while that of non-URM families was $83,332 (95% CI: $79,490–$87,175).

In model 4 we added the variables for SAT scores and ratio, and the variable for the number of family members who are doctors. In this model the only variable with a significant association is family members who are doctors. Female gender no longer has a significant association with the change in level of interest. URM status continues without a significant association. We find no significant association for either individual SAT scores or the ratio of SAT scores. While the explained variance

TABLE 1.3.
Results of least-squares regressions evaluating factors associated with a change
in the level of interest in premedical studies (T3–T1)

	Model 1	Model 2	Model 3	Model 4
URM status	−0.69*	−0.59*	−0.57	−0.07
	(0.31)	(3.30)	(3.32)	(0.36)
Female		−0.74**	−0.74**	−0.50
		(0.74)	(0.27)	(0.28)
Median family income			<0.001	<0.001
			(0.00)	(0.00)
SAT Verbal				−0.002
				(0.02)
SAT Math				0.01
				(0.02)
SAT Ratio (V/M)				4.93
				(15.12)
Number of family members who are doctors				0.33*
				(0.16)
Constant	−0.71***	−1.74***	−1.91***	−11.22
	(0.15)	(0.40)	(0.56)	(15.31)
R-Squared	0.014	0.034	0.027	0.063
F Value	5.13*	6.42**	4.31**	3.35**

Note: T3 = end of sophomore year. T1 = beginning freshman year. Data show regression coefficient (standard error).
***p < .001 **p < .01 *p < .05

(as measured by the value of R-squared) has gone up in model 4 as compared to model 3, the overall fit of the model (as measured by the F value) has gone down. In a separate analysis, we used cross tabulation analysis to determine if (a) URM students and (b) women students tend to report fewer family members as doctors. We found both associations to be significant (data not shown).

The results of our analyses of changes in Stanford students' level of interest suggest three principal findings:

1. Between the beginning of their freshman year and the end of their sophomore year, the premed interest level of URM students declines more than the interest level of non-URM students; this decline is independent of gender.
2. In the same time period, the premed interest level of female students declines more than the interest level of male students; this decline is independent of URM status.
3. Both the number of family members who are doctors (a significant association) and family income (a weak but nonsignificant association) act as inter-

vening variables that replace either URM status or gender as significant predictors of change in level of interest in the models we tested.

Why Do Students Lose Interest?

We learned that, on average, students at both Stanford and UC Berkeley lose interest in continuing premedical studies between the beginning of their freshman year and the end of their sophomore year. The magnitude of the decline is greater at Berkeley than at Stanford. At Stanford we were able to document that the decline in interest disproportionately affects women and URM students. The next question for us was why, in the students' minds, these changes occur. To answer this question, we conducted a series of follow-up interviews at both campuses.

At Stanford we conducted follow-up interviews with 68 of the 362 responding students, administered between the end of the subject's sophomore and senior years. In selecting students for interviews, we attempted to balance students who had reported a decrease in their level of interest in premed with those who had reported an increase in their level of interest. We further divided these two groups into URM and non-URM, then randomly selected students from each group for interview. In doing so, we oversampled URM students.

At Berkeley we conducted one-on-one interviews with 63 of the responding students, also administered between the end of the subject's sophomore and senior years. We divided respondents into two groups, URM and non-URM, and randomly selected students from each group for interview. In doing so, we over-sampled URM students, getting a final interview sample of 29 URM students and 34 non-URM students.

Students had the choice of in-person or phone interviews. In either case, we provided students with the approved consent form (written for in-person, verbal for phone). Each interview was recorded and subsequently transcribed verbatim. A URM interviewer interviewed all URM subjects; a non-URM interviewer interviewed the non-URM subjects.

The interview contained two questions.

1. "What were the factors that led to the [increase] [decrease] in your level of interest in being premed?"

Before finalizing our interview scripts, we had conducted an initial pilot study consisting of informal interviews with several premedical students. In those pilot-study interviews, subjects often mentioned particular courses that they said discouraged their interest in medicine. Based on those preliminary findings, we included question 2 as a follow-up:

2. "Were there any specific courses at [Stanford] [Berkeley] that discouraged your interest in medicine?"

We analyzed data from each of the interview questions separately. For each question, two members of the research team took a sample of the transcripts and closely read the responses in those transcripts. The researchers then discussed these responses in depth. Based on their examination and discussion of this first sample of transcripts, the researchers identified an initial set of response categories. The two team members then took a second set of transcripts, closely read the response in each transcript, and identified response categories in this second sample. This was done to determine whether, and to what extent, the categories in the initial set of categories also represented the data in the second set of transcripts. After this initial coding process with two samples of transcripts, all transcripts (including those in the first two samples) were analyzed using the response categories derived from this process.

Results of Interviews with Stanford Students

As shown in table 1.4, the most frequent response category for the first question was "courses taken at Stanford," mentioned by 36 of the 68 students (53%). (Recall that students were not asked specifically about the influence of courses they had taken until the next question was asked.) The second most frequently mentioned influence was contact with physicians, identified by 13 students (19%).

The way a student reacts to specific courses taken at Stanford as a freshman or sophomore appears to have an important influence on that student's ongoing level of interest in continuing in premedical studies. An especially positive response to those courses will be associated with an increase in interest, while an especially negative response will be associated with a decrease in interest. This contrast is illustrated in the following responses to this question. The first two experienced an increase in interest in premed, and the second two a decrease in interest.

"Information—I took biology at Stanford—the bio core—so understanding the way they actually presented material in medical school curriculum, as well as the topics covered." (URM male, interest level increased)

"The realization that I could handle the academic workload. You hear all those rumors about 'weeder' courses, but I saw that I could do it. I feel I have a decent grasp of what I expect and what is expected of me." (non-URM male, interest level increased)

TABLE I.4.
Comparing by underrepresented minority (URM) status and gender the factors
contributing to a change in interest in being premed as reported during interviews by
self-identified premed students entering Stanford University in 2002, 2003, or 2004

	Increased Level of Interest (N=35)	Decreased Level of Interest (N=33)
URM		
No.	14	10
Reported factors contributing to change in interest	• 5 (36%)[a]—courses taken • 4 (29%)—contact with physicians • 1—advising/adviser • 1—exposure to medical career opportunities • 1—faculty • 1—research	• 7 (70%)—courses taken • 3 (30%)—lost their motivation • 2 (20%)—required too much time/work • 1—advising/adviser • 1—contact with physicians • 1—change in interests
Non-URM		
No.	21	23
Reported factors contributing to change in interest	• 7 (33%)—courses taken • 4 (19%)—contact with physicians • 3 (14%)—research • 1—family member's influence • 1—increased confidence • 1—not interested in any other career • 1—other students' influence	• 17 (74%)—courses taken • 10 (43%)—change in interests • 4 (17%)—contact with physicians • 3 (13%)—family member's influence • 2—advising/adviser • 1—did not want to commit to premed • 1—research
Female		
No.	16	22
Reported factors contributing to change in interest	• 6 (38%)—courses taken • 5 (31%)—contact with physicians • 1—advising/adviser • 1—faculty • 1—not interested in any other career • 1—research	• 19 (86%)—courses taken • 6 (27%)—change in interests • 3 (14%)—lost their motivation • 2—too much time/work • 1—contact with physicians • 1—advising/adviser
Male		
No.	19	11
Reported factors contributing to change in interest	• 6 (32%)—courses taken • 3 (16%)—contact with physicians • 3 (16%)—research • 1—family member's influence • 1—other students • 1—exposure to medical career opportunities • 1—increased confidence	• 5 (45%)—courses taken • 5 (45%)—interests changed • 4 (36%)—contact with physicians • 3 (27%)—family member's influence • 2 (18%)—advising/adviser • 1—research • 1—did not want to commit to premed

[a] Percentages given only for those categories of response with >10%.

"Everyone says it's [Stanford's premed courses] more like a weeding-out process than anything [else] and I just ended up being one of those people." (URM male, interest level decreased)

"I think I experienced the same distaste [as other premeds] for the large premed classes, like the Biology core. You think that no one wants to support you; they're just out to get you." (non-URM female, interest level decreased)

One-third of students whose interest had increased over the period of this study identified courses they took as contributing to that increase, while three-fourths of students whose interest had decreased over the period of this study identified courses they took as contributing to that decrease. The current courses offered to premeds at Stanford appear substantially more likely to discourage students' interest in medicine as a career than to encourage that interest.

Having had contact with a physician during the first two years of college also appears to affect the level of students' interest. In this case, that contact appears more likely to encourage students in maintaining their interest (23%) than to discourage that interest (15%). An exposure to research also seemed to play a role in increasing interest in premed for some students.

It should be noted that among students at Stanford who lost interest in premed, one in three (33%) reported that their interests had simply changed, without identifying a specific contributing factor. It is difficult to know if this change in interest is in reaction to or independent of the other negative experiences reported.

In comparing the responses of URM students with those of non-URM students, the pattern of responses is generally the same. Experience with courses was mentioned most frequently, with those losing interest substantially more likely to mention the effect of courses.

As shown in table 1.5, of the 35 students whose interest in premed increased, 26 (74%) identified at least one course they took during their first two years at Stanford that tended to discourage their interest in a career in medicine. Of the 33 students whose interest in premed decreased, 28 (85%) identified at least one course they took during their first two years at Stanford that tended to discourage their interest in a career in medicine. The responses of URM and non-URM groups were quite similar.

When we then looked to see what specific courses students mentioned as discouraging their interest in medicine, we saw a striking pattern: students identified chemistry courses *between four and five times more often* than the next category, biology. Other courses, such as physics and math, were mentioned only rarely. It is also instructive to note that, among students whose interest in premed had de-

TABLE 1.5.
Specific courses mentioned during interviews by students self-identified as premed entering
Stanford University in 2002, 2003, or 2004, in response to the question, "Were there any
specific courses at Stanford that discouraged your interest in medicine?"

	Increased Level of Interest (N=35)	Decreased Level of Interest (N=33)
URM		
No.	14	10
No. identifying one or more course	11	9
Courses mentioned	• 10 (91%)—chemistry • 4 (36%)—biology • 2 (18%)—physics	• 10 (100%)—chemistry • 2 (20%)—physics • 1 (10%)—mathematics
Non-URM		
No.	21	23
No. identifying one or more course	15	19
Courses mentioned	• 13 (87%)—chemistry • 2 (13%)—biology • 1 (7%)—physics	• 21 (100%)—chemistry • 5 (26%)—biology • 2 (11%)—physics • 1 (5%)—mathematics • 1 (5%)—medical school course
Female		
No.	16	22
No identifying one or more course	13	21
Courses mentioned	• 11 (85%)—chemistry • 3 (23%)—biology • 1 (8%)—physics	• 23 (100%)—chemistry • 3 (14%)—biology • 2 (10%)—physics • 2 (10%)—mathematics
Male		
No.	19	11
No. indentifying one or more course	13	7
Courses mentioned	• 12 (93%)—chemistry • 3 (23%)—biology • 2 (15%)—physics	• 8 (100%)—chemistry • 2 (29%)—biology • 2 (29%)—mathematics • 2 (29%)—physics • 1 (14%)—medical school course

Note: Percentages are based on the number of students who identified at least one course. Some students mentioned more than one course within a category.

creased, students often mentioned more than one chemistry course as having contributed to that decline.

For those students who mentioned at least one chemistry course as having discouraged their interest, we compared the frequency with which specific chemistry courses were mentioned. "Organic chemistry" was the course mentioned most frequently as tending to discourage students' interest in medicine (19/54). "Chemistry" as a generic subject without mentioning a specific course (16/54), and inorganic chemistry (16/54) were each mentioned nearly as often as organic chemistry. Finally, "chemistry lab" was mentioned least often (3/54). These findings confirm those of Lovecchio and Dundes from an earlier study at a single institution.[13] However, our findings suggest that the discouraging effects of studying chemistry as part of the early premedical curriculum are more extensive than organic chemistry alone. The following excerpts from the interview texts are typical of students' responses:

> "*Chem 33 and Chem 36 [both organic chemistry] kinda discouraged me. It was difficult to get a helping hand.*" (non-URM male whose interest level increased)

> "*Organic chemistry.*" (URM male whose interest level increased)

> "*Chem 31 [inorganic chemistry] and Math—first quarter calculus—huge anonymous classes with bad TAs.*" (non-URM female whose interest level decreased)

> "*The chem core, Chem 31/33. It's tough and I think there's a lot of students. There's not a lot of professor-student contact. I felt the professor [was] somewhat abrasive at times.*" (URM female whose interest level decreased)

Results of Interviews with Berkeley Students

As was the case at Stanford, when asked to identify factors that had contributed to the change in their level of interest in premedical studies, Berkeley students most often identified courses they had taken. Students' responses to the question, "Were there any specific courses at Berkeley that discouraged your interest in medicine?" are shown in table 1.6.

As shown on the right side of the table, 28 of 29 URM students (97%) mentioned at least one course that discouraged their interest in medicine. Many of these students mentioned more than one course. By contrast, 22 of the 34 non-URM students (65%) mentioned at least one course as discouraging them.

For those students mentioning more than one course, the interviewer followed up with a question asking the student to identify the one course that was the most discouraging for them. Of the 28 URM students mentioning at least one course, chemistry was cited as the most discouraging course by 20 (71%). Of the 22 non-URM students mentioning at least one course, chemistry was cited as the most discouraging course by 12 (55%). For both groups of students, chemistry was cited *be-*

TABLE 1.6.
List of courses that discouraged students' interest in premedical studies

Most discouraging course			All discouraging courses reported		
Course	URM Students (N=29)	Non-URM Students (N=34)	Course	URM Students (N=29)	Non-URM Students (N=34)
Chemistry (all courses)	20	12	Organic chemistry	11	12
Biology	3	3	Inorganic chemistry	11	4
Math	4	2	Chemistry—unspecified	4	2
Physics	1	3	**Chemistry—total**	**26**	**17**
Interdisciplinary science	0	1	Biology	9	9
Language courses	0	1	Math	11	2
No course discouraged me	1	12	Physics	1	5
			Interdisciplinary science	0	1
			Language courses	0	1
			No course discouraged me	1	12

tween four and five times more often than the next courses, biology and math. It thus seems that, consistent with the results of our interviews with Stanford students, chemistry courses are the single most important factor that discourages students from continuing in premedical studies.

While more than one-third of the non-URM students responded that none of their courses discouraged their interest in premedical studies, only one of the 29 URM students reported this absence of discouraging courses. It appears that chemistry and the other premedical courses at Berkeley are quite a bit more discouraging for URM students than for non-URM students.

Consistent with our concern that many of these URM students, especially those coming from a disadvantaged educational background, may be vulnerable to a loss of self-confidence during the early university experience with a resultant shifting of professional aspirations, we have excerpted from our interviews with six of the URM students at Berkeley specific text that addresses this issue. All six are female. We looked for any mention by the student during the interview of a course that was so discouraging that, as a result of having taken it, the student may have changed his or her aspiration regarding a career in medicine.

SUBJECT I
Q: How would you compare your current level of interest in becoming a physician with the interest you had when you entered as a freshman?
A: I wanted to do it a lot freshmen year, but afterwards I stopped.

Q: What were the factors that led to the decrease in your level of interest?
A: *I didn't think that I could do very well in the chemistry classes. . . . I wanted to be premed when I first got here. But then after the first semester, I stopped. . . . I think a lot of students get scared after Chem IA [inorganic chemistry].*

SUBJECT 2
Q: What were the factors that led to the decrease in your level of interest?
A: *Chemistry. [laughter] Yeah, just the level of competitiveness here. . . . I'm sorry, but chemistry is just—having to take that much and study a lot it's just— I don't like doing that. So it's just like why do that? . . . I've heard many experiences after taking Chem 3 [organic chemistry]. This is just like the peak. You like it or you don't. This is the turnaround point.*

SUBJECT 3
Q: How would you compare your current level of interest in becoming a physician with the interest you had when you entered as a freshman?
A: *It's changed a lot. Yeah, so. When I first came, I wanted to go into health care. And that's what I knew I wanted to do. But then when I started taking the classes, it changed.*
Q: What were the factors that led to the decrease in your level of interest?
A: *Mainly just the classes and the level of difficulty in the classes. I had to repeat Chem IA.*

SUBJECT 4
Q: Were there any specific courses that discouraged your interest in medicine?
A: *I think having to drop Chem IA in the Spring of my first year made me question whether or not I could do it. . . . I really didn't tell anyone because I didn't want to seem stupid. And then when I eventually had to drop it, I remember like I was hiding from certain people because I didn't want them to know. [laughter] . . . So it was just a matter of me not wanting to feel dumb around other people.*

SUBJECT 5
Q: How would you compare your current level of interest in becoming a physician with the interest you had when you entered as a freshman?
A: *Well, my first semester I was in Chem IA and calculus. And it was just like really, really big lectures and a lot of time. And I just felt like I wanted something that was smaller and more focused. . . . A lot of people get scared either before or after O-chem and decide they don't like it [medicine] anymore.*

SUBJECT 6

Q: Were there any specific courses that discouraged your interest in medicine?
A: Chem IA. Introduction to Chemistry or whatever. I took it twice. Um, well once I dropped after the tenth week mainly because on my part I felt that I didn't put enough effort. It just seemed like no matter how hard I tried, I would still probably do bad on the test and stuff like that. . . . That's probably the class at Berkeley that discouraged me from being premed. . . . My friends also felt discouraged . . . They dropped out of their premed pursuit cuz of Chem IA.

Conclusions from Our Research

Among entering students at Stanford who initially are premed, women and under-represented minority students are less likely to maintain their interest in a medical career through four years of schooling. While each factor appears to exert a weakening influence independently, there is an important gender skewing that makes these effects cumulative. While 61 percent of the non-URM students in our study sample were female, 74 percent of URM students (88% of African American students) in our sample were female.

Among freshmen who enter Berkeley with an initial interest in pursuing premedical studies, we also see a clear pattern of a substantial reduction in the strength of that interest by the end of sophomore year. When we compare the Berkeley data to the data from Stanford, we see a substantially sharper decline in interest among Berkeley students. In addition, the decline is seen among all racial/ethnic groups at Berkeley, while at Stanford the decline in interest among white and Asian students was less than that among African American, Latino, or Native American students.

A principal cause of the decline in interest among premedical students seems readily apparent. Based on the results of our interviews, early experiences in the premedical science courses are frequently reported as having discouraged a student's interest in continuing in premedical studies, with chemistry courses as the principal source of that discouragement. The discouraging effects of chemistry courses appear to be felt more acutely by URM students at both Berkeley and Stanford.

From the results of our interviews, it appears that the adverse effects of chemistry courses experienced by many of the URM students led directly to their questioning their own ability to continue to pursue a medical career and as a consequence dropping medicine as a possible career choice. At both Berkeley and Stanford, a majority of these URM students are women. For these students, entering college with the hope of becoming a physician and then having a negative experience in a chemistry course is a major turning point in their lives. In the words of one of the Berkeley students whose interview appears above, "I'm sorry, but chemistry is just . . . just like the peak. You like it or you don't. This is the turnaround point."

In our interviews with them, a number of Stanford students used the term "weeder course" to describe their experience in the chemistry classroom. Students perceive success in chemistry as essential to gaining admission to medical school. Perhaps the impact of this perception is best summarized by the Stanford URM student quoted above who said, "Everyone says it's more like a weeding-out process than anything, and I just ended up being one of those people."

Questioning the Orthodoxy of Premedical Education

At Stanford University and to a large extent at the University of California, Berkeley, incoming freshmen who aspire to become physicians face substantial pressure to enter the standard premedical curriculum early in their college careers. In most cases this means enrolling in freshman chemistry, followed in sequence by courses in biology and physics. Those who delay this process rapidly become aware that they are, in their own words, "off-track"—that they face a competitive disadvantage among their premedical peers in getting ready to apply to medical school.

As a result of including courses in chemistry in their early academic experiences, many of these students become discouraged, often giving up on their aspirations. We know that two groups of students are more likely to respond to their early experiences in the chemistry classroom by losing interest in a medical career: women and underrepresented minority students. The outcome of this sorting process is that these two universities, two of the most competitive in the country, contribute far fewer URM physicians to the American medical profession than they might.

In 2006 Dr. Ezekiel Emanuel, chair of the Department of Bioethics at the Clinical Center of the National Institutes of Health, published an article in *JAMA* questioning our continued reliance on the traditional premedical curriculum with its heavy emphasis on science courses. Dr. Emanuel suggested that "many premed requirements are irrelevant to future medical education and practice." He went on to argue, "Why are calculus, organic chemistry, and physics still premed requirements? Mainly to 'weed out' students. Surely, it would be better to require challenging courses on topics germane to medical practice, research, or administration to assess the quality of prospective medical students, rather than irrelevant material."[14] By suggesting that calculus, organic chemistry, and physics are "irrelevant to future medical education," Emanuel was challenging what has come to be the orthodoxy of premedical education.

To appreciate how widespread this orthodoxy has become, it is instructive to examine the Web site of the Princeton Review, a private firm that offers premedical students support in preparing for medical school in the form of books, classes, and private tutoring. On its Web site, the review advises students interested in going to medical school to complete one year of biology, one year of inorganic chemistry, one year of organic chemistry, one year of physics (all sciences with accompanying labs), and one year of English.[15] Wikipedia, the increasingly important on-line source of common knowledge, offers advice that is essentially the same.[16] At least for some of the most popular on-line sources of information regarding expectations for premedical students, there is general agreement that the road to medical school begins in the science classroom, and that every premedical student is well advised to take two years of chemistry, one year of biology, and one year of physics.

To confirm the consistency of this expectation among medical schools, I reviewed the minimum requirements for admission as listed on the Web sites of six of the leading medical schools in the country, each (as we will see later in this book) with an important historic role in the evolution of both medical education and premedical education:

- College of Physicians and Surgeons of Columbia University[17]
- Harvard University School of Medicine[18]
- Johns Hopkins University School of Medicine[19]
- University of California, San Francisco School of Medicine[20]
- University of Michigan School of Medicine[21]
- Stanford University School of Medicine[22]

While the schools approach the issue of English and math somewhat differently, each agrees that in order to gain admission premedical students must have completed two years of chemistry, one year of biology, and one year of physics.

The AAMC is explicit in describing what is expected of premedical students at most of its member schools:

> The study and practice of medicine are based on modern concepts in biology, chemistry, and physics, and on an appreciation of the scientific method. Hence, mastery of these basic scientific principles is expected of all entering medical students. Medical schools typically require successful completion of one academic year . . . of biology and physics and one academic year each of general chemistry and organic chemistry. . . . All science courses should include adequate laboratory experience.[23]

If nearly all medical schools agree on the necessity of two years of chemistry, one year of physics, and one year of biology as the minimum acceptable preparation for entry into medical school, when and where was this norm established? Using information published by the AAMC, we find that these standards were set more than fifty years ago.

In 1950, the AAMC first published its *Admission Requirements of American Medical Colleges*. Looking at the 1951 issue of that handbook, we see that the six medical schools listed above all had substantially the same admission requirements in 1951 as they did in 2008.[24] In 1951 they each listed two years of chemistry, a year of physics, and a year of biology as required for admission. Three of the schools wanted a semester of embryology in addition to the required year of biology. However, in 1951 they were unanimous on the need for the same basic science courses—chemistry, physics, and biology—that they required in 2008. For premedical students hoping to gain admission to these medical schools in 1951, as for students today, success in these sciences defines the orthodoxy of premedical education.

Apparently it was also the orthodoxy in 1924, when Sinclair Lewis wrote about his fictional premedical student, Martin Arrowsmith, for whom "the purpose of life was chemistry and physics and the prospect of biology next year."[25]

It thus appears that, in his comments above suggesting that many of the standard premedical requirements are "irrelevant to future medical education and practice" and are there "mainly to 'weed out' students," Ezekiel Emanuel was voicing a somewhat unorthodox view of premedical education. That this is so is reflected in some of the published responses to his remarks.[26] Dr. Daniel Kramer, of Massachusetts General Hospital, responded to Emanuel's assertions by arguing in support of organic chemistry: "I would not so hastily dismiss organic chemistry as a mere tool to thin the applicant herd. Indeed, I believe that no other premedical course so directly impacts clinical practice. . . . I remember very little about benzene rings, but the critical thinking and problem-solving skills of organic chemistry formed the foundation of my medical training." Kramer appears to be arguing that it is not so much the specific knowledge base gained in the undergraduate study of organic chemistry that matters as it is the introduction to organic chemistry as a way of thinking and of reasoning.

Kramer's argument is supported by that of Drs. Thomas Higgins and Scott Reed, surgeons from Eastern Virginia Medical School: "The value of organic chemistry and physics may be difficult to appreciate because medical care does not directly require remembering physics formulas or analyzing chemical structures; however, these disciplines contribute a great deal to providing the framework for understanding basic principles of medicine."

Not all the writers, however, were so critical of Emanuel's unorthodox recommendations. Dr. Virginia Collins and her colleagues from the American College of Physicians respond in their letter that "current premedical requirements reflect tradition rather than any particular educational rationale."

In looking for the origins of our current understanding about what is orthodox and what is unorthodox in premedical education, one might well turn to the Flexner Report, published in 1910 and commonly understood to be a major contributor to the scientific revolution in medical education that took place in the United States in the early part of the twentieth century. There Flexner said of premedical education: "The normal rhythm of physiologic function must remain a riddle to students who cannot think and speak in biological, chemical, and physical language."[27]

What was the basis of Flexner's assertion? Was there scientific evidence to support his view? Did our current model of premedical education develop as a product of sound scientific reasoning, or might it simply have evolved based on a common set of beliefs? What is the empirical evidence that courses in chemistry, physics, and biology are fundamentally necessary to understanding the scientific reasoning on which the practice of medicine is based? It is crucially important to address these questions to be able fully to understand the implications of the current model of premedical education not only for the future ethnic diversity of the medical profession but also for its future intellectual diversity. I will address each of these questions in the following chapters.

CHAPTER TWO

The Historical Origins of Premedical Education in the United States, 1873–1905

In order to trace the origins of premedical education in this country, I have reviewed the history of the premedical requirements established by Columbia University College of Physicians and Surgeons (originally known as King's College, founded in 1767); Harvard Medical School (founded in 1783); University of Michigan Medical School (founded in 1850); Johns Hopkins School of Medicine (founded in 1893); Stanford University School of Medicine (founded in 1908); and University of California, San Francisco School of Medicine (founded in 1873).[1] These schools represent a range of public and private universities; each has made a contribution to the evolution of premedical education.

It is in 1873, with the founding of the University of California, San Francisco (UCSF) medical school, that I begin my study of the history of premedical education. In 1873 neither Harvard nor Columbia listed any prerequisites for admission in their bulletins. Only Michigan had explicit admission requirements, described in the university's bulletin for 1873 in the following terms:

> Every candidate for admission shall exhibit to the Faculty satisfactory evidence of a good moral and intellectual character; a good English education, including a proper knowledge of the English language, and a respectable acquaintance with its literature, and with the Art of Composition; a fair knowledge of the Natural Sciences, and at least of the more elementary mathematics, including the chief elements of Algebra and Geometry, and such a knowledge of the Latin language as will enable him to read current prescriptions, and appreciate the technical language of the Natural Sciences and of Medicine.

The University of California received its original legislative charter in 1868, charged by the legislature with creating first a College of Arts and Letters, followed by a College of Medicine and other professional colleges. In 1872 the university hired as its second president Daniel Coit Gilman, at that time a professor of geography at Yale University and secretary of Yale's Sheffield Scientific School. As described by historian Gert Breiger, "Gilman had already been involved in the planning and beginning of the first premedical course while he was still at Yale, and he was much involved in the consideration of what constituted proper medical education while he was the President of the University of California."[2]

In 1872 there were two medical schools in San Francisco: the Medical College of the Pacific (later to be re-named the Cooper Medical College), originally founded in 1858 by Dr. Elias Cooper; and the Toland Medical College, founded in 1864 by Dr. Hugh Toland.[3] Each was hospital based; neither had an affiliation with a university. Both schools were open to essentially any student able to pay the required tuition. As a result of some unfriendly competition between the two schools and some back-and-forth movement of faculty, Dr. Toland decided it would be best to affiliate his medical school with the fledgling University of California. A series of negotiations ensued, and in March 1873 the trustees of the Toland Medical College deeded their school to the University of California. The Archives of the Library of the University of California, San Francisco, contain a complete collection of the bulletins of the medical school, starting with the first bulletin published in 1875. A review of these bulletins indicates that there were no specific admissions requirements listed for the new medical school.

Building on his years at Yale, President Gilman worked to incorporate a vigorous education in the natural sciences as part of both the medical education provided at the new medical school and the expected preparation for entry into medical school. Gilman argued, "Chemistry, zoology, comparative anatomy, these should all be thoroughly learned before the student takes up medical studies."[4] Dr. Ronald Fishbein, former admissions dean at the Johns Hopkins School of Medicine, describes Gilman's efforts to inculcate in the minds of the leaders of the new university and of the medical profession in California the importance of a medical education grounded in the sciences:

> He spoke of "those branches of knowledge which lie at the foundation of medicine." He pointed out that students enter medical school where "they learn for the first time that there are such sciences as physics, chemistry, and physiology, and are introduced to anatomy as a new thing." He proposed that the educational system be adjusted to make available the elements of physical sciences to those who were preparing for the further study of medicine. He felt that these subjects should be conquered before acceptance into medical school.[5]

However, Gilman was not successful in getting the University of California to adopt preparation in the sciences as a prerequisite for entry into the university's medical school. The leaders of the university viewed Gilman's emphasis on a rigorous preparation in the natural sciences as somewhat unorthodox by the then-extant standards. Failing to gain support for his approach to medical and premedical education, Gilman left the University of California in 1875 to become the first president of the newly established Johns Hopkins University. Not until 1885 would UCSF establish as a specific requirement for admission "a matriculation examination . . . in the following subjects: English; Arithmetic; Geography; Elementary Chemistry."

While Gilman may not have been fully successful in California, he nonetheless did have a substantial impact on the future of medical education. As described by Fishbein, Gilman's effort, "was one of the first public pronouncements of a trend in scientific medical education that would eventually engulf American universities and medical schools."[6]

Contemporaneous with Gilman's efforts to imbue medical education at the University of California with a scientific foundation were those of Charles W. Eliot toward that same end at Harvard. Despite considerable faculty opposition like that faced by Gilman, Eliot was to be substantially more successful over time. An 1853 graduate of Harvard, Eliot had traveled to Europe to study both the rapidly evolving field of chemistry and European systems of higher education. While in Europe, he had closely observed the German system of medical education in which, as described by Paul Starr, "the laboratory sciences of physiology, chemistry, histology, pathological anatomy, and somewhat later, bacteriology were revolutionizing medicine."[7]

Whereas in England, and subsequently in the United States, instruction in medicine had historically been provided either on the apprenticeship model or in medical schools based in hospitals, medical education in Germany was largely the responsibility of universities. In the mid-nineteenth century when sciences such as chemistry, physics, and physiology began to expand the breadth and depth of knowledge, it was in close proximity and close cooperation with the clinical faculty. As natural science expanded in laboratories of the German university, medical science expanded accordingly.[8]

Germany had also established a system of secondary education based on the Gymnasium, a rigorous secondary school in which the best students prepared for potential entry into the university. Those completing the Gymnasium took a series of examinations, with students passing the exams eligible to enter the university. Upon matriculating at the university, a student could select from among the available curricula, one of which was medicine. Typically, there was little if any chemistry, biology, or physics taught in the *Gymnasium*—students received instruction in these sciences as part of the university-based medical curriculum.

Both Eliot and Gilman proposed that medical education in the United States should adopt the German model, but with one important difference. They agreed that medical schools should be based in universities; however, both felt that sciences such as chemistry, biology, and physics should be taught as part of the undergraduate curriculum in preparation for medical school rather than being included as part of the medical curriculum.

In 1865 Eliot returned to the United States to take a position as professor of chemistry at MIT. He was committed to the concept that medical education should be the responsibility of universities and that it should be based on an early and rigorous education in the basic sciences, especially chemistry. Four years later, when he assumed the presidency at Harvard, he turned his attention both to reforming the nature of undergraduate education there and to reforming medical education. As described by Kenneth Ludmerer, Eliot "was convinced of the importance of science to medicine and of the need to teach scientific principles with laboratories as well as with lectures."[9] Ludmerer goes on to quote Eliot's comments from his first report as president of Harvard, presented in 1870 at a time when only 20 percent of Harvard medical students had a college degree: "The whole system of medical education in this country needs thorough reformation. The ignorance and general incompetency of the average graduate of American Medical Schools, at the time when he receives the degree which turns him loose upon the community, is something horrible to contemplate."[10]

Eliot proposed a fundamental series of reforms for the medical school. One of the first was that, as university president, he also assumed the role of chair of the medical faculty. Then, in 1871, he introduced three fundamental reforms to the medical school: (1) the medical school became an integral part of the university; (2) the length of the medical school course was extended from two years to three, with mandatory examinations at the end of each year; and (3) the course of medical instruction would be based on first acquiring education in the basic sciences, with heavy use of the laboratory as part of the instruction.[11]

The changes in Harvard's system of medical education initiated by Eliot in 1871 are also reflected in changes to the entrance requirements to the medical school. Recall that in 1873 there were no published requirements for entry into Harvard's medical school. In 1875 the first statement of prerequisites appeared:

In and after September, 1877, all students seeking admission to the Medical School, must present a degree in Letters or Science from a recognized college or scientific school, or pass examinations in the following subjects:

- Latin (French or German will be accepted, however, as a substitute for Latin)
- Physics.

In the Medical School Bulletin of 1877 this requirement was amended with the addition of the following: "All candidates for admission, except those who have passed an examination for admission to Harvard College, must present a degree." In Germany and France it was the norm that all students completing the European equivalent of high school were required to pass a rigorous examination before entering the university. Once in the university, students were free to select from available courses of study, including medicine. Because most medical students at Harvard had had, at most, only a high school education, Eliot wanted to be sure that both students entering Harvard College as undergraduates and students entering the Harvard Medical School had had an adequate high school education. For the medical school this entailed as a minimum a knowledge of physics and of either Latin, French, or German. Entering students were not initially expected to have had a course in chemistry. That subject was part of the early curriculum within the medical school.

In 1880 the list of subjects to be covered by the medical school's entrance examination was expanded to include English, Latin, physics, and "any one of the following subjects: French, German, Algebra, Plane Geometry, or Botany." In 1893 a required examination in chemistry was added to the list, and the following statement appeared: "Candidates who present a degree in Arts, Literature, Philosophy, or Science from a recognized college or scientific school are exempt from all of the above examinations, with the exception of Chemistry."

Concurrent with the extension in 1892 of the medical school's required curriculum from three years to four, an explicit expectation was established that entering medical students will have had a course in chemistry. Students who had graduated from a college other than Harvard and who wanted to attend the Harvard Medical School were exempted from all entrance examinations with the exception of that in chemistry. It appears that Eliot was giving predominance to the science in which he was originally trained.

While Charles Eliot was working to strengthen the scientific grounding of medical education at Harvard, Daniel Coit Gilman was working at Johns Hopkins University to accomplish the same thing. Johns Hopkins University was founded in 1876, with Gilman selected as its first president. The university had been created by the bequest of Johns Hopkins, a leading member of the Quaker community in Baltimore. Before his death in 1873, Mr. Hopkins had explicitly stated that he wished his legacy to be used to found a university, a hospital, and a medical school. These were the tasks assigned to Gilman when he took charge of Johns Hopkins. Gilman worked hard to attain these goals, and in 1889 the hospital was opened. As described later in this chapter, the medical school would not be ready to open until 1893, and only after a complex series of negotiations between President Gilman, the university trustees, and a group of feminists from Baltimore.

From the outset, Gilman was clear about the direction he wanted the medical school to take. The university's curricular bulletin from 1877 described what Gilman considered to be the optimal preparation for the study of medicine: "Physics, Chemistry, and Biology, with Latin, German, French, English form the principal elements of this course."[12] In making his recommendations, Gilman had relied heavily on advice he had received from several leading medical educators in Europe, among them Charles Huxley and Henry Acland of England and Joseph Lister of Scotland. Based on his own perspective and the advice of these noted scholars, in 1878 Gilman submitted a report to the Johns Hopkins trustees titled "On the Studies Which Should Precede a Course of Study in Medicine, Hygiene, Etc." In his report, Gilman argued, "First, a standard of admission to medical colleges should be agreed upon, and every respectable institution should insist on a real, and not a pro forma examination to be passed by every matriculant . . . there is in our present circumstances no other method by which suitable candidates for the medical profession can be chosen, and the unsuitable eliminated."[13] In Gilman's 1878 remarks we see the first explicit indication of the need to use the sciences to eliminate —to weed out—those candidates who are unsuitable for entry to medical school. Later in the report Gilman describes in some detail the "Programme of Studies preparatory to medical studies" that a student at Johns Hopkins would be expected to follow:

> He will have followed for a year . . . a course of instruction in Natural Philosophy [a common way at that time to refer to the study of physics] and will have had the opportunity of working with scientific instruments in the physical laboratory during the same period.
>
> He will have attended for a year a course of lectures, examinations, and demonstrations in Chemistry, and will have worked in the chemical laboratory four hours daily, during a year and a half.
>
> In Biology he will have worked for a considerable part of two years, and will have pursued a thorough course of dissection and demonstrations both in comparative and human anatomy, and in physiology.
>
> He will have a good command of English, and will have been taught Latin, French, and German. He will read at sight ordinary books in the languages last named.

We see in Gilman's proposed premedical curriculum the first explicit roots of the premedical curriculum faced by students today. What Gilman proposed in 1878 was most certainly not the orthodoxy of premedical education at that time. No other medical school in the United States had come close to establishing such a rigorous premedical curriculum. Recall that in 1878 Harvard expected only a high school education, with examinations required in Latin and physics. In 1878 Columbia listed no entry requirements.

At that time there were also two young organizations working in support of Gilman's and Eliot's approach to strengthening medical education and its scientific foundations. In 1876, representatives of twenty-two medical schools had convened in Chicago in order "to consider all matters relating to reform in medical college work."[14] They agreed to establish a new organization, which they named the American Medical College Association. The assembled delegates agreed to establish a common policy regarding the minimum requirements of a medical education. Among these requirements were a minimum of three years study under the direction of a "'regular' graduate and licentiate and practitioner of medicine" (medical educators at that time had begun to differentiate between "regular" medical practitioners and "irregular" practitioners), and a requirement that every student shall also have "matriculated at some affiliate college or colleges, for two regular sessions," and during those two sessions will have studied and passed an examination in a list of subjects that included chemistry and physiology. At their meeting in 1880, the delegates voted to extend to three years the minimum course of study in a medical college.

While the delegates who founded the organization and established these requirements were enthusiastic in their efforts, the general response to those efforts was less than enthusiastic. After establishing the three-year requirement, membership in the association began to dwindle. A number of medical schools were unwilling to adopt these heightened expectations. At the 1881 meeting of the association, only eighteen schools sent delegates; in 1882 the number of delegates was eleven. No further meetings of the fledgling organization were held. As described by Dean F. Smiley, in 1957 secretary of the Association of American Medical Colleges, "The Association was dead. The new organization had tried to raise standards too rapidly."[15]

In 1890 representatives from several medical schools in Baltimore (the Johns Hopkins medical school had not yet been established) issued a proposal to reconvene the association, and a series of preliminary meetings was held. Delegates to these meetings voted to reestablish the organization and to rename it the Association of American Medical Colleges (AAMC). By that time the general sentiment had shifted regarding the wisdom of establishing national standards of medical education, and the renamed organization was able to grow in both number of schools represented and national influence. The new role of the association is described later in this chapter.

In 1876, the same year that the ill-fated American Medical College Association was founded, a second group of medical educators met to establish a parallel organization, the American Academy of Medicine (AAM). As described by historian Steven Peitzman, the AAM was "a society formed largely by literary minded small town doctors concerned that medical students knew no Latin or Greek . . . locally recognized well-educated physicians, many residing in small towns, not . . . giants of the profession."[16] The members of the AAM had all been to college before studying medicine. It was their purpose to "encourage young men to pursue regular courses of study in classical, scientific, and literary schools of the highest grade, before entering upon the study of medicine." The constitution of the AAM recognized two categories of members: Fellows, and Honorary Members. To be accepted into the academy:

> The Fellows shall be Alumni of respectable institutions of learning, having received therefrom—
>
> (1) The degree of Bachelor of Arts, or Master of Arts, after a systematic course of study, preparatory and collegiate;
>
> (2) The degree of Doctor of Medicine, after a regular course of study, not less than three years.[17]

The AAM had called for the same three-year course of study as had the American Medical College Association. However, the AAM was largely an association of individuals, not of medical schools, so the failure of most medical schools to adopt their standards did not dampen their enthusiasm. The AAM continued to meet regularly throughout the 1870s and 1880s. In 1891 it began to publish the *Bulletin of the American Academy of Medicine*. Beginning in 1893 the *Bulletin* began to publish the proceedings of the AAMC and for several years was its official publication. The AAM also established a close working relationship with the National Conference of State Medical Examination and Licensing Boards. The early years of the *Bulletin* contain many references to joint efforts between that organization, the AAM, and the AAMC to get laws passed in the various states restricting the issuance of licenses to practice medicine only to graduates of medical schools that met the standards adopted by these organizations. For several years these three organizations held their annual meetings together. The American Medical Association joined those efforts in 1905.

The early volumes of the *Bulletin* of the AAM contain a series of very interesting papers, addressing the issue of what type of preliminary education should be expected of medical students. One of the first was by David Starr Jordan, an 1875 graduate of Indiana Medical College and president of the University of Indiana. Shortly after giving his address to the annual meeting of the AAM in 1891, Jordan took a new job as the first president of a newly established university in California, the Leland Stanford Junior University. In 1908 Jordan was to preside over the founding of the Stanford School of Medicine.

In his paper to the AAM titled "The General Education of the Physician," Jordan supports the basic precepts of the AAM, saying: "The Bachelor's Degree as generally understood is an index of general culture, the gauge of that degree of training which fairly prepares a bright young man to enter upon professional work."[18] Jordan notes, though, that by requiring a bachelor's degree before beginning the study of medicine, the student "is not through college and ready to begin his professional studies much before the age of twenty-two." He acknowledges that many medical schools consider this lengthy preparatory period to be unreasonable, with many students unable to begin the practice of medicine much before the age of twenty-six or twenty-seven. "Is the standard of the Bachelor's degree too high for the best results in professional work?" Jordan asks. "In other words is the physician who has waited to secure his Bachelor's degree thereby handicapped in his professional life? . . . I cannot think so, and I am sure that no such view could be sustained by statistics."[19] He goes on to argue that the undergraduate premedical course should include the study of chemistry, physics, physiology, and a reading knowledge of German and French. Jordan cites the premedical curriculum that had been established by Johns Hopkins University as consistent with these expectations. That curriculum was to become a prerequisite to admission when the Johns Hopkins Medical School opened two years later in 1893.

In his 1892 presidential address to the AAM, Dr. P. S. Conner argued that chemistry should be taught, not as part of the medical course, but as an undergraduate subject that is preparatory to medical education: "Chemistry in the didactic medical course is a non-essential of the first order, and the hours devoted to it [in medical school] are simply wasted. . . . No one should be permitted to enter on the study of medicine who has not at least an ordinary school-boy acquaintance with the elements and their compounds. . . . If . . . the undergraduate would have an extended, more thorough course in organic and animal Chemistry, by all means give him the opportunity."[20]

A paper presented to the annual meeting of the AAM in 1892 described the premedical course at the University of Pennsylvania,[21] which approached chemistry and physics as well as Latin, Greek, French, and German as subjects to be taken as an undergraduate before beginning the study of medicine. Dr. Helen Warner from

Detroit then rose to speak in response to the paper describing Pennsylvania's curriculum. "Chemical training," she commented, "while it is more useful in one sense, at least more directly productive, is less educative to the whole man than the more general literary training. So it is that a man may be a wise and intelligent physician, or a very skillful surgeon, and have never learned to express himself clearly and to the point, or to write good plain English without rhetorical effusion."[22] Dr. Warner's comments about the disjuncture between knowledge of chemistry and verbal ability presage arguments and research results that would only appear more than a hundred years later. As it turns out, and as we will see in chapter 4, when the Standardized Patient Examination was added to the series of tests required for medical licensure in the United States, a student's verbal ability was found to be a better predictor of clinical skills than was knowledge of chemistry.

In 1893 Victor C. Vaughan addressed the AAM. A practicing physician with a special interest in toxicological chemistry, Vaughn had become dean of the University of Michigan Medical School in 1891. The previous year, Michigan had lengthened its required medical school course from three years to four and had established the requirement that those not having a high school diploma must pass a series of examinations that included physics, biology, and Latin.

While supporting the need for a broad undergraduate education as preparatory for the study of medicine, Vaughan is clear on the need to include an in-depth study of science as part of the premedical curriculum.

> He who would practice the profession in the best light of today must make himself familiar with the sciences which contribute to medicine and with the best methods of applying the facts thus ascertained. . . . The medical man must be familiar with physics in its various branches . . . ; with chemistry, both inorganic and organic; with botany, microscopy, hygiene, bacteriology, physiology. . . . Lacking knowledge in any one of these sciences, the medical man is constantly limited and crippled in his work.[23]

Vaughan went on to state that the study of these sciences must include extensive work in the science laboratory. In an earlier paper, Vaughan had suggested that medical students should spend at least four hours per day in the laboratory as part of their study of chemistry, biology, and physics.[24]

With the addresses given by Conner in 1892 and Vaughan in 1893, we are beginning to see an important shift in the dominant approach to premedical education. There was a growing consensus that chemistry, physics, and biology should be part of undergraduate premedical education. In addition, we begin to see the argument that the study of chemistry should be extended to include both inorganic chemistry and organic chemistry. What was unorthodox when Gilman had proposed it in 1873 and again in 1878 was becoming mainstream in 1892.

In 1893 Harvard began to require entering medical students to pass examinations in English, Latin, physics, and chemistry, although students could have taken these courses either in high school or in college. By that time the University of California, San Francisco, had a similar requirement, requiring entrance examinations in English, arithmetic, geography, physics, and chemistry. Michigan would accept either a high school diploma or examinations in these subjects in lieu of a diploma.

The situation in 1893 at Columbia, however, is instructive. For the first time, the following statement appeared in the bulletin of the medical school: "To all persons who matriculate with the intention of becoming candidates for the degree of doctor of medicine *at any school in the State of New York,* the following provisions of law are now applicable, viz.: Laws of New York, 1893, Chapter 661, ¶ 145 (in part)." In 1893 a law had been passed in New York, delegating to the Regents of the University of the State of New York the task of giving those students who wished to enter medical school anywhere in the state a "medical-student certificate." Without this certificate, a student could not enter the medical school at Columbia. According to an earlier law passed in 1889, in order to obtain that certificate a student must have completed "a full year's course of study in any college or university under the supervision of the Regents" and passed an examination in "arithmetic, grammar, geography, orthography, American history, English composition, and the elements of natural philosophy."

For more than a decade, organizations such as the AAM and the National Conference of State Medical Examination and Licensing Boards had been advocating for laws defining standards both for medical education and for premedical education. They were successful in getting such a law approved in New York, and Columbia began following their requirements. The new standards of premedical education had been elevated from a growing consensus to a matter of law, at least in New York.

The Founding of the Johns Hopkins School of Medicine, 1893

As described above, Daniel Coit Gilman, president of Johns Hopkins University, had addressed the trustees of the university in 1878 regarding his views on the standards of premedical education. Under this "Programme of Studies," a premedical student "must study here for three years or more and pass numerous examinations. A large part of his time will be passed in the laboratories of Physics, Chemistry, and Physiology."[25] In discussing what undergraduate degree these students would receive from Hopkins after they had completed this course of studies, Gilman remarked to the trustees, "One gentleman has playfully suggested that if we were not fettered by traditional initials [such as B.A., B.S.], the degree of F.S.M., 'fit to study medicine,' would tell the tale exactly."[26] Gilman again seems to be suggesting that it is at the undergraduate level that students should be sorted into those who are fit to study medicine and those who are not.

Gilman was successful in establishing a formal premedical curriculum at Johns Hopkins. Referred to as the "Chemical-Biological course," this was what we recognize today as an undergraduate major. As described in the first Johns Hopkins Medical School catalogue issued in 1894, this course "is planned for the professional education of those students who have been especially fitted to receive its instructions by a course of preliminary training in the liberal arts, and especially in those branches of science, like physics, chemistry, and biology, which underlie the medical sciences." When the medical school first opened in 1893, only those students who had completed this course at Hopkins or an equivalent course at another college or university were eligible for admission. By requiring both a bachelor's degree and a rigorous course of university-level sciences, Johns Hopkins established a standard of premedical education that in 1893 was unique in the United States. However, the story of how Gilman and Hopkins came to this requirement is somewhat more complex and involves others who were working to define new standards of higher education.

In September 1885, Bryn Mawr College was first opened as a Quaker college for women. Its first dean was M. Carey Thomas, a 28-year-old scholar of languages, the first woman ever to be awarded a Ph.D. summa cum laude from the University of Zurich. Born and raised in Baltimore, Thomas had a series of relatives and family who served as trustees of both Bryn Mawr College and Johns Hopkins University. As an indication of the close link between the two schools, Daniel Coit Gilman was one of the speakers at the inaugural ceremonies for Bryn Mawr. Gilman had previously consulted with Thomas in the planning for Bryn Mawr, encouraging her to strengthen the college's offering in the sciences.[27]

Thomas had overcome a series of obstacles to attaining her doctorate, not the least of which were the explicit rules prohibiting women from enrolling at many American universities. After graduating from Cornell, she had been permitted to begin graduate studies at Johns Hopkins but had been limited to individual consultations with her graduate advisor. At that time women were not allowed to attend the doctoral seminars that were the core of doctoral education at Hopkins. She was forced to travel to Europe to complete her doctoral work, again encountering gender bias that delayed her completing her degree. It was only when she transferred to the University of Zurich that she was successful in completing and defending her thesis.

While in Europe, Thomas became thoroughly versed in the German system of higher education. Never a medical student herself, she nonetheless had ample opportunity to observe the German system of medical education that Gilman at Hopkins, Eliot at Harvard, and Vaughan at Michigan were using as the basis of their own reforms. It was her hope that Bryn Mawr would develop both a world-class undergraduate college for women and a program of graduate education equal to that of Europe.

Thomas had developed an extremely close circle of women friends in Baltimore, many of whom were also the daughters of trustees of either Bryn Mawr or Johns Hopkins. One friend in particular was to play a major role in the opening of the Johns Hopkins medical school—Mary Garrett, the daughter of John Work Garrett, president of the Baltimore and Ohio Railroad and one of the richest and most influential men in Baltimore. Like Leland Stanford and his Central Pacific Railroad, John Garrett used his influence and wealth to support the establishment and expansion of institutions of higher education. As described by historian Helen Lefkowitz Horowitz, Mary Garrett and Carey Thomas had a relationship that was both emotionally close and physically intimate. Garrett, who had inherited substantial personal wealth from her parents, used that wealth to further Thomas's career at Bryn Mawr. In 1893 Garrett had pledged a substantial donation to the college on the condition that they name Thomas as president, a step to which the trustees eventually acceded.[28]

Daniel Coit Gilman had been working for several years to carry out the wishes of Johns Hopkins, the original benefactor of the university that bore his name. After successfully opening the university itself, Gilman next worked with the trustees to found a hospital, a step he helped to complete in 1889. He then turned his attention to the opening of a medical school.

Shortly before the hospital was opened, Mary Garrett approached Gilman with a proposition: she would commit to raising $100,000 in support of the new medical school if the Hopkins trustees would agree to admit women on an equal footing with men once the school opened. Garrett had seen the difficulties Carey Thomas had faced in her own graduate work at Johns Hopkins. She would use her money and her influence to open medical education at Hopkins to women. She founded the Women's Medical School Fund, calling on wealthy and influential women she knew throughout the United States to contribute to it. By 1890 she had raised the money, and the Hopkins trustees agreed to her request. From its very first day, the Johns Hopkins Medical School would be open to women as well as to men.

Hesitant to overcommit the university's endowment, however, the trustees established the policy that the medical school would only open once a new endowment of $500,000 could be raised. Garrett's gift would count toward that amount, but Gilman still needed to raise an additional $400,000. By the end of 1892, Gilman had made little progress in raising this amount. This gave Thomas and Garrett an opportunity to have even more influence in setting the direction for the new medical school.

Thomas, based on her experiences in Germany and Switzerland, wanted the medical school at Johns Hopkins to be founded and operated on the principles common to the German model of medical education. After a series of letters and conversations between Thomas and Garrett, on December 24, 1892, the Hopkins trustees were presented with a letter from Mary Garrett containing a new offer.[29] She would commit to fully funding the required endowment, including a gift of more than $300,000 from her own funds, thereby enabling the opening of the medical school. She would do so, however, if and only if the Hopkins trustees agreed to the following conditions:

1. The new medical school would include a minimum four year course for the medical students;
2. The school would accept only those students who had completed the requirements for a Bachelor's Degree, either at Johns Hopkins or at another approved college or university;
3. To be eligible for admission to the medical school, students were required to complete as part of their undergraduate education a course of study equivalent to the prescribed premedical course at Johns Hopkins, which included:
   a. One year of physics, with three hours per week of laboratory instruction;
   b. One year of chemistry, with five hours per week of laboratory instruction;
   c. One year of biology, with five hours per week of laboratory instruction;
4. All students would have a good reading knowledge of French and German.

In addition, Garrett insisted that if at any time in the future the Johns Hopkins Medical School violated these conditions by changing either the length of the medical school curriculum or the premedical admission requirements, the entire endowment would be transferred to Bryn Mawr College. She described the reasoning behind her proposal in the following terms: "These stipulations and, in particular, those relating to the standard of admission, instruction and graduation in the medical school, I make not because of any misgiving in regard to the policy likely to be pursued by the present board of trustees, but because of the obvious possibility that the policy might be altered by succeeding trustees."[30]

Gilman was in an interesting bind. For twenty years he had argued for extending and strengthening the scientific foundation of both the medical school curriculum and the premedical curriculum. Now he had a major donor insisting that Johns Hopkins establish the most stringent premedical requirements of any school in the country and commit to maintaining those requirements in perpetuity. The requirements suggested by Thomas to Garrett and required by Garrett as a condition of her funding the endowment of the medical school contain essentially the same requirements medical students face today. A reading knowledge of German and French is no longer required; however, the requirement that a student complete courses in physics, chemistry, and biology is still at the core of premedical requirements in the United States today.

On January 3, 1893, ten days after the trustees had received Garret's proposal, Gilman spoke to the Hopkins trustees at a meeting called to discuss the Garrett offer. He cautioned the trustees: "These conditions, we must remember, are prescribed not for a year or a term of years but for all time."[31] Gilman was extremely reluctant to lock the trustees into requiring a specific premedical curriculum because, as he saw it, "changes which no one can foresee will in time be required by the progress of knowledge and the improvement of educational methods." In addition, Gilman was concerned that "it is not easy to foresee by what test our medical faculty can ascertain whether other kindred courses of undergraduate study are equivalent to those that are here prescribed [i.e., the established premedical curriculum at Johns Hopkins]."

As we will see in the following chapter, Gilman was justified in his concern. Over time the chemistry requirement would need to be lengthened from one year to two years to encompass the burgeoning field of organic chemistry. In addition, as English became the predominant language of the medical literature, a reading knowledge of German and French became less and less relevant to medical education and medical practice. Toward the end of the twentieth century this requirement would be dropped at Johns Hopkins (a move that required the consent of the Bryn Mawr trustees, since it was a technical violation of the original Garrett grant).

Gilman and Garrett had a series of discussions in which Gilman suggested that the premedical requirement be described as "a long course of preliminary training in the liberal arts and especially in those branches of science like Physics, Chemistry, and Biology which underlie the medical sciences." Garrett and Gilman agreed to include a statement in their legal agreement that the conditions laid down by Garrett "shall not be construed as restricting the liberty of the University to make such changes in the requirements for admission to the Medical School of the Johns Hopkins University . . . as shall not lower the standard of admission specified in this clause."[32] To monitor and enforce this agreement and the conditions it established, the trustees agreed to publish the terms of the agreement yearly in the university's bulletin and to establish a Women's Committee of the Medical School, "to whom the women studying in the Medical School may apply for advice concerning lodging and other practical matters."[33] Included on this committee were Mary Garrett and M. Carey Thomas.

Garrett and the trustees came to a final agreement on February 20, 1893, two days before the university's previously scheduled celebration of its Commemoration Day. At the commemoration ceremony, Gilman gave a speech announcing the opening of the Johns Hopkins Medical School, with the first students enrolling in the fall of that year. In that speech Gilman traced the history of the efforts to establish the medical school from the founding of the university in 1876. He described the evolution of the premedical requirements he had worked to establish at Hopkins:

> In Baltimore, a distinct course of studies (in which physics, chemistry, and biology, with the modern languages, were dominant) intended to be preparation for the subsequent study of medicine, was arranged and offered to students . . . as early as 1878. . . . [I]t has remained upon our register, with hardly any changes, awaiting the time to come when the organization of a medical school and the enlistment of additional teachers should give both the impulse and the opportunity to prune and graft our promising vines, so that in the future they may bear more fruit than leaves.[34]

In grafting a vine from one rootstock to another so that it may flourish and grow, a gardener selects the healthiest shoots, trimming and discarding those with less promise. After his unsuccessful attempt at the University of California, Gilman was finally successful (with the help of M. Carey Thomas and Mary Garrett) in establishing the premedical curriculum he believed in and in using students' performance in that curriculum to identify those who are "Fit to Study Medicine," pruning and discarding those who are not.

Growing Support for the Standardization of Premedical Education, 1893–1905

The years following the opening of the Johns Hopkins Medical School saw a rapid coalescing of both interests and organizations in support of the models established at Johns Hopkins for both medical education and premedical education. At the annual meeting of the Association of American Medical Colleges in 1894, a resolution was passed requiring member schools to extend their medical curriculum to a min-

imum of fours years.[35] In 1901 the AAMC published its list of the premedical requirements that member schools were expected to require. These included examinations in English, math, physics, and Latin.[36] (In 1901 the AAMC required an examination in physics but not chemistry, while in that same year Harvard, with
chemist Charles Eliot at the helm, required a bachelor's degree and an examination
in chemistry but not in physics.)

The year 1901 saw another important change that was to have profound effects
on the course of medical education and premedical education. The American Medical Association (AMA), first established in 1847, underwent a fundamental reorganization, with centralization of its authority under a House of Delegates, a board
of trustees, and executive officers. As described by Morris Fishbein, who from 1924
until 1950 was editor of the *Journal of the American Medical Association,* as a result
of this reorganization, "the basic structure of the Association was placed on a firm
footing."[37] One of the first actions of the new president of the organization was to
appoint a Committee on Medical Education "to survey the problem of medical education in this country and make recommendations concerning the role which the
American Medical Association should play in the improvement of medical education."[38]

Chaired by Arthur Dean Bevan of Rush Medical College in Chicago, the committee reported back to the House of Delegates in 1903 with a list of recommended
policies, which included:

That it is desirable that a uniform and elevated standard of requirements for
the degree M.D. should be adopted by all the medical schools in the United
States;
  That it is desirable that young men before being received as students of medicine should have acquired a suitable preliminary education.[39]

A year later, Bevan reported back with a more strident commentary and a specific
recommendation for future action:

In absence of national governmental control efforts to make uniform and elevated
the standard of medical education can be made most effective through the agency
of the organized medical profession of the entire country, and such a body we now
have in the reorganized American Medical Association.
  The problem of using to the best purpose the weight and influence of the
American Medical Association toward elevating medical education is a very large
one and one which must be carefully worked out. This can best be done by a permanent committee or council specially created for this purpose.[40]

In response to Bevan's report, the House of Delegates voted to create a Council on Medical Education (CME) with the charge "to act as the agent of the American Medical Association (under instruction from the House of Delegates) in its efforts to elevate medical education."[41] The delegates appointed Bevan as chair of the CME and named four additional members, one of whom was Victor C. Vaughan of Michigan. As dean of the medical school at Michigan, Vaughan had served in 1902–1903 as president of the AAMC. In his address to that organization at the end of his term, Vaughan had stated clearly his position and the position supported by the AAMC regarding the standard of premedical education that should be applied: "At present the average graduate of the average . . . high school has an inadequate preparation in the modern languages and in the natural sciences. I mean by this that in these branches he is not, in my opinion, prepared for the study of medicine, and he should be required to pursue these subjects in some well-equipped academy, college, or university before he enters the medical school."[42]

At the time Vaughan made these remarks, the State of Michigan had passed a law that mandated defined premedical requirements for entry into any medical school in Michigan, much as New York had done earlier. The Michigan medical school itself required two years of college, with courses in physics, biology, and chemistry and a reading knowledge of either German or French. Thus, the appointment of Vaughan to the Council on Medical Education and his appointment as chair of the CME's Committee on Requirements for Admission to Medical Schools were a clear indication of the direction the CME intended to take regarding premedical education.

Coincident with the creation of the CME in 1904, George H. Simmons, recently appointed as secretary of the AMA and editor of the *Journal of the American Medical Association,* published a speech he had given earlier that year. In it Simmons argued, "It is essential to fix a minimum below which no medical college should be allowed to admit students." He went on to refer to the opening of the Johns Hopkins Medical School, citing "the startling announcement that the requirements for admission would be, not only a bachelor's degree in art, but also a year's work in biology, physics, and chemistry and a reading knowledge of French and German." Simmons suggested that "it is too Utopian to imagine that the minimum requirement for entrance to the professional school shall be the full college course." Instead, he proposed that the minimum entrance requirement be set at two years of college, which would provide "a general knowledge of biology, of chemistry, of physics, of electricity, of light and sound. These are necessary—absolutely so." However, he went on to qualify his recommendation with the following statement: "I refer to *a thorough mastery of the fundamentals, not the mere acquisition of such chemical facts* as may seem from time to time, with the progress of our science, to be directly applicable to its practice and teachings" (emphasis added).[43]

Following the charge given to it, the CME organized a national conference on medical education, held in Chicago in April 1905. In his introductory remarks to this conference, Dr. Lewis McMurtry, president of the American Medical Association, described the purpose of the meeting as "bringing together the various examining and licensing powers of the states and territories, to secure a mutual interchange of ideas and counsel."[44] In addition to delegates from several of the state licensing boards, the AAMC was also represented at the meeting.

Arthur Bevan, chair of the CME, summarized for the conference the view of the five-member council:

> What would be regarded as a perfectly satisfactory state of affairs for medical education, we might say ideal state of affairs, from our perspective view-point? Such medical education must be equal to that required by England and Germany. It would comprise:
>
> 1. A preliminary education such as would enable the student to enter our standard universities . . .
> 2. Five years of medical work, the first year to include physics, chemistry, and biology. This year either to be taken in a medical school or in a college of liberal arts.[45]

Two of the delegates to the conference—Prof. Richard D. Harlan of Lake Forest College and Dr. J. M. Dodson from the AAMC—suggested that adding introductory courses in chemistry, physics, and biology to the medical school curriculum would make that curriculum too crowded. Instead they suggested, as described by Dr. Dodson, "eliminating [from the medical school curriculum] such subjects as chemistry, physics, and general biology, which can be taught to better advantage in colleges of liberal arts."[46] There appeared to be general consensus at the conference that the teaching of these basic sciences was best left to the undergraduate institutions rather than being added to the curriculum of the medical schools.

Victor C. Vaughan then reported on the activities of the CME's Committee on Requirements for Admission to Medical Schools, of which he was chair. Speaking to the requirement of a reading knowledge of German and French (the standard set by Johns Hopkins in 1893), Vaughan reported, "We would not say that a reading knowledge of German and French should be required for admission to all our medical schools, but it certainly should be recommended and those schools which can require it should do so." Vaughan then summarized the admission requirements recommended by his committee, which included "the fundamental facts of physics, chemistry, and general biology" supplemented by laboratory instruction in these subjects.[47]

During his comments, Vaughan also urged "the enactment of laws taking the decision on preliminary requirements out of the hands of the medical faculties and placing it on official boards."[48] George Simmons, secretary of the AMA, concurred with Vaughan's suggestion and urged the AMA to establish a close working relationship with the state licensing boards throughout the country. In reporting to the AMA's House of Delegates on the CME's inaugural conference, Arthur Bevan described as the "ideal standard" the four-year course of medical education the delegates to the conference had identified, preceded by a year studying physics, chemistry, and biology. He recommended to the delegates that they adopt this model as AMA policy and work "to secure the general adoption of these requirements by state boards and medical schools."[49] The House of Delegates enthusiastically agreed, approving the CME's recommendation.

The AMA had aligned itself with the AAMC and with the leaders of the most prestigious medical schools in the country. A new standard of medical education was adopted, involving two years of instruction in laboratory sciences followed by two years of instruction in clinical practice. This four-year medical school curriculum would be preceded by one or two years in the study of physics, chemistry, and biology in a college or university. Discussing these new standards, Morris Fishbein stated, "In the light of present-day [1947] requirements, they seem modest. In 1905, they represented a marked advance."[50]

What was unorthodox when Gilman proposed it in 1878 had become the new orthodoxy in 1905. Thus it was that when Martin Arrowsmith had been a premedical student in 1904, "The purpose of life was chemistry and physics and the prospect of biology next year."[51]

CHAPTER THREE

A National Standard
for Premedical Education

Between 1893, with the opening of the Johns Hopkins Medical School, and 1905, with the actions of the inaugural conference of the Council on Medical Education (CME), there was a remarkable coalescing of interests in the United States around a single national standard for both medical education and premedical education. This coalescence is reflected in the premedical admission requirements of the medical schools we have been following. In 1893, all the schools except Johns Hopkins had required only a high school diploma and examinations in a range of subjects. In 1905, Johns Hopkins and Harvard both required a bachelor's degree. While Hopkins required undergraduate courses in chemistry, biology, and physics, Harvard required only an undergraduate course in chemistry, though recommending courses in the other sciences. The Universities of Michigan and California required two years of college, with courses in the three natural sciences. Columbia deferred to the requirements set by the State Regents, which specified one year of college and examination in a range of subjects that included chemistry, biology, and physics.

The work of the American Academy of Medicine (AAM), the Association of American Medical Colleges (AAMC), and the American Medical Association (AMA) had been effective in creating a coalition to argue and lobby for the application of these standards nationally. By 1905 they had been successful in getting several states to pass laws that limited the granting of a medical license to graduates of medical schools that adhered to the standard of medical education and premedical education promulgated by these organizations. As has been noted, New York and Michigan were among the states that had passed such laws. California passed a law in 1901 that was to have a direct influence on the founding of the Stanford University Medical School in 1908.

The Founding of a New Medical School in California
and the Closing of an Old One, 1901–1908

In 1873 there were two principal medical schools in San Francisco. That year the Toland Medical College had transferred its assets to the recently created University of California, leaving the Medical College of the Pacific as the principal private medical school.

The Medical College of the Pacific had been founded in 1858 by Dr. Elias Cooper as the first medical school on the Pacific Coast. Between 1873 and 1900, the school was reasonably successful, changing its name to the Cooper Medical College in honor of its founder.[1] With a substantial endowment donated by Dr. Levi Cooper Lane, a successful surgeon and the nephew of the founder, the college had acquired a medical school building and a successful hospital. As the benefactor of the school and as the leader of its faculty, Dr. Lane had kept abreast of the movement to elevate and standardize medical and premedical education. In the 1890s he had extended the school's curriculum to four years and established the requirement of a high school diploma for admission, largely in response to the standards published by the AAMC. As Dr. John Wilson explained in his history of the Stanford Medical School:

> With respect to the critical issue of admission standards, which ultimately determine the quality of the profession, the Faculty was well aware that Presidents Eliot of Harvard, Gilman of Hopkins and Jordan of Stanford all advised that a bachelor's degree or its equivalent should ultimately be required for entrance to medical school. Nevertheless, the Faculty was unprepared to take such a step. Like other free-standing proprietary schools, Cooper College depended upon tuition for its support. High standards for admission would have resulted in a disastrous reduction in the student body and in tuition income. It was growing increasingly clear to the Directors and Faculty of the College that only financial underwriting by a parent body such as a university could provide for the higher admission standard called for by the presidential triumvirate.[2]

However, the faculty of Cooper Medical College faced a problem. In making the initial financial bequest that permitted the college to acquire the building for its school and the affiliated hospital, Dr. Lane had stipulated, "This College shall never be affiliated with, or become the department of any other educational institution, but shall remain an independent school in which Medicine and its Kindred Sciences shall be taught."[3] While the financial viability of the college depended on affiliating with a university in order to be able to raise its admission standards to meet the evolving AAMC requirements, Dr. Lane's bequest prohibited such an affiliation.

On February 27, 1901, the California legislature passed a law titled, "An act for the regulation of the practice of medicine and surgery in the State of California, and for the appointment of a board of medical examiners in the matter of said regulation."[4] The efforts of the AAM, the AAMC, and the National Conference of State

Medical Examination and Licensing Boards described in the previous chapter had come to fruition in California. The state had created a board of medical examiners and delegated to the Medical Society of the State California (the state affiliate of the AMA) the authority to name a majority of the board's members. The law specified that in order to be eligible for a license to practice medicine in California a physician must possess "a diploma issued by some legally chartered medical school, the requirements of which medical school shall have been at the time of granting such diploma, in no particular less than those prescribed by the Association of American Medical Colleges for that year."[5]

In 1901 the AAMC published the following statement of its requirements for admission to a medical school: "Each college holding membership in this Association shall require of each student, *before admission* to its course of study, an examination, the minimum of which shall be as follows . . ."[6] The statement then went on to list the specific content expected in English, arithmetic, algebra, physics, and Latin. (There was no mention of chemistry or biology.) The statement also indicated that, in lieu of the examination, member colleges "are at liberty to recognize the official *certificates of reputable* literary and scientific colleges, academies, high schools, and normal schools."[7]

Dr. Lane was fully aware of the direction the AAMC was taking in defining premedical requirements. He had changed the medical school curriculum and the admission requirements at Cooper Medical College to conform to the 1901 standard, but he realized that the college would have substantial difficulty maintaining these requirements over time while also remaining financially viable. Wilson's history of the Stanford Medical School reports, "In January 1902, during the last weeks of a terminal illness characterized chiefly by progressive exhaustion and anxiety, Dr. Lane decided to revoke the pledge. By this time he had accepted the view that medical schools in the United States were destined to be integral parts of universities."[8] He also urged the remaining directors of the medical school to consider affiliating with Stanford University, which had been founded a decade earlier by the railroad magnate Leland Stanford.

In September 1902, Clarence John Blake, an eminent ear surgeon from the Harvard Medical School, wrote to David Starr Jordan, president of Stanford, encouraging him to consider establishing a medical school through an affiliation with Cooper Medical College. In the letter Blake first argues the general point that a medical school should be part of a university: "The day of the private venture in medical education in this country is fast drawing to a close and the main outlook for the advance of medical education is the medical school, not chartered to members of the medical profession nor established as the adjunct to a hospital, but created as an integral part of the university system."[9] Blake then goes on to point out, "An examination of the plant of the Cooper Medical College shows it to be available for the purpose of a university hospital," and he encourages Jordan to take advantage of "the wealth of clinical material within your reach" by merging with Cooper.

In the years immediately following Dr. Lane's death, there appear to have been few serious discussions between the leaders of the Cooper Medical College and President Jordan of Stanford regarding a possible merger. The leaders of Cooper worked to establish a medical library in memory of Dr. Lane and continued to run the medical school in a manner that largely followed the requirements laid down by the AAMC. Then, on April 18, 1906, San Francisco experienced a major earthquake and fire that destroyed much of the city. While the school's Lane Hospital was not severely damaged, the school nonetheless experienced a major disruption: "The net result was marked temporary loss of patient income which, in addition to costly building repairs, put a serious strain on the budget of the College. It was of special significance that the disaster occurred at a time when income from student fees was declining and annual budget shortfalls were beginning to occur. These circumstances heightened the interest of the Directors in a liaison with Stanford."[10]

Dr. C. N. Ellinwood was at that time president of Cooper Medical College. Faced with the financial disruptions of the earthquake on top of the pressures of adhering to the AAMC's standards as was required by law, Ellinwood approached Stanford about a possible merger. He appointed a committee of Cooper faculty to carry out these discussions. On August 1, 1906, the Stanford University trustees also appointed a committee to negotiate with Cooper about a possible merger. That committee reported back to the trustees on November 1, recommending that Stanford "maintain a department of medicine on a basis of scholarship and efficiency equal to that of the very best medical schools in the country."[11]

Stanford University had first opened in the fall of 1891. Its First Annual Register for the 1891/92 school year states, "Students intending to enter on the study of medicine, will take Physiology and Histology as a major subject, with collateral work in Chemistry, Botany, and other sciences."[12] By the 1894/95 school year, that statement had been expanded to read: "Students intending to enter on the study of medicine, are advised to take Physiology and Histology as a major subject, with Chemistry, Physics, Comparative Anatomy of the Vertebrates, and Hygiene among the collateral subjects. Such a course gives that foundation both in scientific knowledge and in skill in experimental Physiology, and in Histological and Anatomical technique, which will make it possible to accomplish the medical course of the best medical schools in a much shorter time and with much greater advantage."[13]

Recall that, as described in the previous chapter, President Jordan had addressed the AAM in 1891, arguing in support of the requirement of a bachelor's degree as a prerequisite for admission to medical school. Even before Stanford was to establish its medical school, Jordan had introduced to Stanford an undergraduate premedical major modeled closely on the premedical major created by Daniel Coit Gilman at Johns Hopkins.

A series of detailed negotiations took place, and on September 14, 1907, President Jordan reported to the trustees, "I have reached the conclusion that it is wise for Stanford University to accept the offer recently made by the Cooper Medical College." Jordan went on to say, "The degree of MD should not be granted in less than seven years from the date of matriculation in the freshman class."[14]

The recommended premedical major at Stanford as described in the bulletin for 1907–08 is essentially the same as that published in 1894–95. Thus it was clear that, should Stanford establish a medical school, it would include admissions requirements that were essentially the same of those at Johns Hopkins. This is precisely what happened. The Stanford trustees approved Jordan's recommendation, and in 1908 the Stanford Medical School accepted its first class. As reported by President Jordan in his Annual Report for 1908, and as stated in the University's bulletin for the 1908–1909 school year, "Three years of collegiate work in Stanford University, or its equivalent as accepted by the Committee on Advanced Standing, will be required for admission to the course in Medicine. This preparatory course must include one year of Physics with laboratory work, one year of Chemistry with laboratory work, one year of Physiology or Biology with laboratory work, and French or German (such a reading knowledge as shall be acceptable to the Department of Medicine)."[15]

The legal requirement facing Cooper Medical College as a result of the state law passed in 1901, coupled with the devastation of the 1906 San Francisco earthquake, apparently placed an insurmountable burden on the leaders of the college. With David Starr Jordan as its president, Stanford University was to replace Cooper with its own medical school. In doing so, Stanford closely followed the example set by President Gilman of Johns Hopkins and acted in full support of and compliance with the national standards described in 1905 by the CME.

The CME Standards and the Flexner Report, 1905–1910

The CME and the AAMC worked in close collaboration to support the extension of the standards identified in 1905. When Arthur Bevan retired from the CME in 1928, he described the activities of the CME after 1905 in a speech to the AMA's Annual Congress on Medical Education, Medical Licensure, and Hospitals: "As the Council continued to study the problem, it soon became evident that the most important piece of work to be done by the Council was to make a personal inspection of the more than 160 schools; to ascertain the character of their plants, of their work and of their faculties, and in general their fitness to teach medicine; and to mark them as one might in giving a civil service examination."[16]

As described by Dr. Bevan, members of the CME personally visited each of the schools in the country, grading them on such factors as the curriculum, physical plant, laboratory facilities, hospital facilities, and policies regarding admission requirements. Schools were graded on a 100–point scale and, based on this grading, divided into three groups:

- Class A—schools scoring above 70 points, labeled as "acceptable"
- Class B—schools scoring from 50 to 70 points, labeled as "doubtful"
- Class C—schools scoring below 50 points, labeled as "nonacceptable"

These inspections, completed in 1907, yielded the following results:

- 82 (51%) were rated as Class A
- 46 (29%) were rated as Class B
- 32 (20%) were rated as Class C[17]

Many of the schools in the lower category were schools of homeopathic medicine or "eclectic" medicine that did not adhere to the scientific standards promulgated by the CME and the AAMC. "It early became apparent," said Bevan in his 1928 address, "that as soon as the one-year, and then the two-year university requirement of physics, chemistry and biology was generally adopted, homeopathy and eclecticism would die for lack of students, and this proved to be the case."[18]

The CME had evidence of the shortcomings of many of the medical schools in the country, yet did not yet have a public forum or base of public support broad enough to translate those findings into new public policy. Bevan explained in 1928,

> As the work of the Council developed, it occurred to some of the members of the Council that, if we could obtain the publication and approval of our work by the Carnegie Foundation for the Advancement of Teaching, it would assist materially in securing the results we were attempting to bring about. With this in mind we approached President Henry S. Pritchett of the Carnegie Foundation, presented to him the evidence we had accumulated and asked him to make it the subject of a special report on medical education by the Carnegie Foundation. He enthusiastically agreed to this proposition.[19]

The Carnegie Foundation for the Advancement of Teaching (Carnegie Foundation) was founded in 1905, the same year the CME held its inaugural conference. Henry Pritchett, its first president, was an astronomer who, like many of the leaders in medical education, had studied in Germany. Like those leaders, he became enamored of the German model of science and science education—thus his enthusiasm for accepting the CME's proposal to repeat their study. In his history of U.S. medical education, Kenneth Ludmerer describes the relationship between CME and the Carnegie Foundation:

> Since it seemed politically imprudent for a medical organization to be so publicly critical of medical schools, the council invited the Carnegie Foundation for the Advancement of Teaching to conduct a similar study, and Henry Pritchett, the president of the Carnegie Foundation, readily accepted the invitation. Records of both the council and the Carnegie Foundation indicate how closely the two cooperated in performing the survey. As a political stratagem, however, it was decided not to make public the council's role in organizing the study. . . . Thus, the report could be publicly perceived as the independent judgment of an outside agency.[20]

Pritchett attended the 1908 meeting of the CME to discuss further the idea of the Carnegie Foundation's picking up where the CME had left off. The minutes of that meeting reflect the understanding between Pritchett and Bevan, and between the Carnegie Foundation and the CME: "[Pritchett] agreed with the opinion previously expressed by the members of the Council that while the Foundation would be guided very largely by the Council's investigation, to avoid the usual claims of partiality no more mention should be made in the report of the Council than any other source of information. The report would therefore be, and have the weight of an independent report of a disinterested body, which would then be published far and wide. It would do much to develop public opinion."[21]

Pritchett selected Abraham Flexner to conduct the study for the Carnegie Foundation. Flexner had graduated from Johns Hopkins in 1886, earning his bachelor's degree in only two years by passing out of some required courses and double-booking his academic schedule. As he described in his autobiography, he had to enlist the personal intervention of President Gilman to permit him to take make-up exams when he found that the double-booked courses had scheduled their final exams at the same time.[22]

After receiving his degree from Johns Hopkins, Flexner moved to Louisville, Kentucky, and at the age of nineteen became a high school teacher. He eventually started his own private high school, which enjoyed considerable success. After nearly twenty years as a high school teacher, now married and with a young child, Flexner spent an evening sitting with his wife, thinking about their future. When his wife asked him, "What would you do if you had never married?" Flexner replied, "I should quit schoolteaching and go to Europe." "Then that is what we will do," his wife replied, and their life took an entirely different turn.[23] In 1905 they closed down the school and pooled their savings, a sum that would allow him to spend a year taking graduate courses in psychology and philosophy at Harvard and then a year touring Europe, engaged in an independent study of the European educational system.

Flexner returned from Europe in 1907. His savings largely exhausted, he began looking for work. He consulted with Ira Remsen, Daniel Coit Gilman's successor as president of Johns Hopkins University. Gilman had left Johns Hopkins in 1902 to become, at the request of Andrew Carnegie, the first president of the Carnegie Institution of Washington (currently the Carnegie Institution for Science). Flexner requested from Remsen a letter of introduction to Henry Pritchett, the former president of M.I.T., whom Andrew Carnegie had asked to become the president of the recently established Carnegie Foundation for the Advancement of Teaching. Pritchett offered Flexner the position as lead researcher on the study of U.S. medical schools.

According to Ludmerer, "It is well known how little Flexner knew about medicine as he began the project in December 1908."[24] In Flexner's own words describing his initial response to Pritchett's offer, "As our family resources had been depleted during the preceding three years I was, I confess, prepared to do almost anything of a scholarly nature. . . . I called his attention to the fact that I was not a medical man and had never had my foot inside a medical school."[25] Pritchett offered Flexner the job nevertheless.

In preparing for the study, Flexner read extensively and traveled to Chicago "for two reasons: first, to confer on the general situation in medical education with Dr. George Simmons, secretary of the American Medical Association . . . ; second, to read the reports prepared for the Council on Medical Education of the association by Dr. N. P. Colwell."[26] He also traveled to Baltimore to meet with the leadership of the Johns Hopkins Medical School. Flexner was later to comment, "The rest of my study of medical education was little more than an amplification of what I had learned during my initial visit to Baltimore."[27] Flexner decided to use the model of the Johns Hopkins Medical School as the metric with which to evaluate the other medical schools in the country: "I had a tremendous advantage in the fact that I became thus intimately acquainted with a small but ideal medical school embodying in a novel way, adapted to the American conditions, the best features of medical education in England, France, and Germany. Without this pattern in the back of my mind, I could have accomplished little. With it I began a swift tour of medical schools in the United States and Canada—155 in number, every one of which I visited."[28]

Working closely with Dr. Colwell, secretary of the CME, Flexner visited these schools, using an analytic framework similar to that used by Colwell in the CME study and using the Johns Hopkins model as the frame of reference. Apparently, Colwell accompanied Flexner on a number of his medical school visits, although the actual number of joint visits remains unclear. In his 2002 biography of Flexner, Thomas Bonner comments that Flexner gave somewhat conflicting descriptions of how often he and Colwell traveled together as part of the study, sometimes reporting that he and Colwell "made many trips together," and other times suggesting that the number of joint trips "could hardly have exceeded half a dozen."[29] Flexner has described his methodology in the following terms:

> In half an hour or less I could sample the credentials of the students filed in the dean's office, ascertain the matriculation requirements . . . , and determine whether or not the standards . . . set forth in the school catalogue were being evaded or enforced. A few inquiries made clear whether the faculty was composed of local doctors . . . or the extent to which efforts had been made to obtain teachers properly trained elsewhere. A single question elicited the income of the medical school. . . . A stroll through the laboratories disclosed the presence or absence of apparatus, museum specimens, library, and students. . . . Finally, the situation as respects clinical facilities was readily clarified by a few questions. . . . In the course of a few hours a reliable estimate could be made respecting the possibilities of teaching modern medicine in almost any one of the 155 schools I visited.[30]

Flexner completed his assigned task in eighteen months. The Carnegie Foundation published the results of his study, titled *Medical Education in the United States and Canada: A Report to the Carnegie Foundation for the Advancement of Teaching*, in 1910. That report has come to be known simply as The Flexner Report. While the bulk of the report focused on medical education and the need to reduce the number of medical schools, Flexner is quite explicit in the report about the standards of premedical education that should be adopted by American medical schools. Early in the report Flexner asks "how much education or intelligence it requires to establish a reasonable presumption of fitness to undertake the study of medicine under present circumstances."[31] Flexner's comment, by which he frames the issue of premedical education, is notable for two reasons. The first is what might be interpreted as equating education with intelligence. He seems to be suggesting that the extent to which a premedical student has succeeded in studying the sciences as an under-graduate is a reflection of the student's inherent intellectual ability and thus can be used as an accurate gauge of the ability to succeed in medical school and as a physician. The second is his use of essentially the same wording to describe the role of premedical education as Daniel Coit Gilman had used in 1878 when he described the role of premedical education as determining which students are "F.S.M.—fit to study medicine." Here Flexner describes the role of premedical education as identifying those students with "a fitness to undertake the study of medicine." Flexner's conception of the role and content of premedical education seems to have been heavily influenced by Gilman's earlier work. In his autobiography, Flexner wrote, "Those who know something of my work long after Gilman's day, at the Carnegie Foundation . . . will recognize Gilman's influence in all I have done or tried to do."[32]

Flexner goes on in his 1910 report to answer his own question about the prerequisites for medical education when he states: "The normal rhythm of physiologic function must then remain a riddle to students who cannot think and speak in biological, chemical, and physical language. . . . [A]dmission to a really modern medical school must at the very least depend on a competent knowledge of chemistry, biology, and physics. Every departure from this basis is at the expense of medical training itself. . . . We have concluded that a two-year college training, in which the sciences are 'featured,' is the minimum basis upon which the modern medicine can be successfully taught."[33]

Flexner is breaking no new ground in his description of the "minimum basis" of premedical education as involving two years of college with courses in chemistry, biology, and physics. As described in the previous chapter, these were precisely the requirements adopted by the CME and the AAMC in 1905. While in 1905 there had been some discussion of the need for one year of college versus two as sufficient to complete the required courses in the sciences, by 1910 the consensus was that two years was the necessary minimum. In 1910 each of the six medical schools we have been following required at least two years of college with courses in chemistry, biology, and physics. Flexner was simply restating what had already become the new orthodoxy of premedical education.

There is another important aspect of Flexner's analysis of premedical education that warrants discussion. Despite his report being about the importance of science as the basis of medical knowledge and medical practice, he offers no scientific evidence to support his claims regarding "the minimum basis upon which the modern medicine can be successfully taught." To state emphatically that "the normal rhythm of physiologic function must then remain a riddle" to students who had not successfully completed the specific premedical curriculum he describes, without offering sound evidence in support of his claim, is to ask the reader to accept as scientific fact what was instead the evolving system of beliefs regarding premedical education. While researchers in Flexner's era may have considered Flexner's compilation of descriptive data to be scientific, in reading his report today we quickly see how little scientific evidence it actually contains. Rather than a scientifically established association, his assertion regarding medicine remaining a "riddle" to those who had not studied the required sciences reflected his own belief and that of those he had relied on for advice.

It is important to appreciate that those who adhere to an orthodoxy often view their belief as having the weight of scientific truth. By modern research standards, though, Flexner conducted his study with substantial bias built into its methodology, using superficial data gathered "in the course of a few hours." His claim that his research results presented "a reliable estimate" of the ability of the medical schools to provide an adequate medical education is open to question.

Regardless of the scientific accuracy of all its claims, the Flexner Report was to have a profound effect on medical education in the United States. Fifteen thousand copies were printed and distributed, and "newspapers accepted it as gospel."[34] Both public opinion and the laws governing the practice of medicine in the various states turned against the schools that had not adopted Flexner's model of medical education and premedical education. Both the number of medical schools in the country and the number of schools not following the CME/AAMC precepts were reduced dramatically.[35] In the 1906 study conducted by the CME there were 160 medical schools nationally, of which 78 (49%) did not meet the CME/AAMC standard. When the survey was repeated in 1915, there were only 95 medical schools still in operation, of which 29 (31%) did not meet the standard. In 1920 only 15 of the remaining 85 schools (18%) did not meet the standard.

In February 1914 the CME convened its Tenth Annual Conference. In his chairman's address, Arthur Bevan reported on the progress the CME had made since first defining its standard of medical education and premedical education in 1905: "For the last nine years the Council on Medical Education and this conference have worked steadily and untiringly to bring about the adoption of this standard, and they have succeeded so far that this general adoption is now clearly in sight. . . . Then no state licensing board required more than a high-school education; now sixteen state boards require one or two years of college work, including courses in physics, chemistry, and biology." Bevan went on to argue that "medicine has become not only a function of the state, but one of the most important functions of the state."[36] It seems clear that Bevan was relying on close collaboration among the

CME, the AAMC, and the National Conference of State Medical Examination and Licensing Boards to apply the force of law to the educational standard they had developed.

Victor C. Vaughan of Michigan also addressed the 1914 CME conference, restating in somewhat more vehement terms the position he had argued earlier: "No man is fit to study medicine, unless he is acquainted, and pretty thoroughly acquainted, with the fundamental facts in physical, chemical, and biological subjects. . . . The facts of the biological, physical, and chemical sciences are the pabulum on which medicine feeds. Without these sciences, everything that goes under the name of medicine is fraud, sham and superstition."[37] If chemistry, biology, and physics were the premedical orthodoxy of the time, Victor C. Vaughan was one of the leading supporters of that orthodoxy.

The 1914 meeting of the CME heard a dissenting voice, however. After forty years as president of Harvard University, Charles W. Eliot stepped down and in 1909 was replaced by A. Lawrence Lowell. Lowell had graduated from Harvard Law School in 1880 and had entered the practice of law. In 1898 he joined the Harvard faculty as a professor of government. He had no training or first-hand experience with medical education or premedical education. Speaking to the CME in 1914, he expressed skepticism about the premedical standard they had adopted: "It would be presumptuous in me to question the validity of medical opinion on the content of the necessary premedical education, but one may properly inquire how well the rules adopted by this association are fitted to attain the object sought, and *how far they may have the effect of excluding able men from the profession*" (emphasis added).[38]

Lowell went on to argue against expecting college freshmen to focus on completing their premedical requirements early in their college career at the expense of their broader education. From Lowell's perspective, it would be preferable to have students use their early college years to strengthen their general academic abilities and then to tackle the premedical courses as college seniors, something they could do more efficiently and more effectively at the end of their college careers: "A college education which has any value in training the mind must make men more capable of grappling with difficult subjects than they were before, and, consequently, must fit them to acquire mastery of a subject more rapidly than before they went to college. If so, a man ought to learn a certain amount of physics, chemistry or biology in a shorter period and with less hours of lectures and laboratory work in his senior year than in his freshman year."[39]

Lowell points out that a standard course in the sciences taken in the freshman year would qualify a student for admission to medical school, whereas a shorter, more focused course taken as a senior would not. "In short, you are requiring not a result but a process; you are ascertaining not whether the man has a proper preparation for the study of medicine, but whether he has gone through a régime of training which may in ordinary cases secure the result desired, but which is sometimes not necessary for the purposes, and often inadequate."[40]

Lowell does not appear to be rejecting the "ideal standard" of premedical education, but rather he seems to suggest that it should be one of multiple options in preparing for medical school. Some students may do well taking their premedical sciences early in their college career; some may do equally well avoiding the sciences until their senior year, instead focusing their early college years on acquiring a broad educational base for the subsequent study of medicine. By requiring the former, students who might do better with the latter are often excluded from medicine as a career.

Lowell goes on to cite statistics he had gathered at Harvard and published in 1911, which we will examine in more detail in the following chapter. Using as his measure of success the percentage of students who graduated from Harvard Medical School with cum laude honors, Lowell summarized his findings by concluding "that a large amount of scientific preparation is not an essential, or indeed a highly important preparation for medical studies, and that a small amount is not a hindrance to successful work. . . . [F]or the study of medicine, excellence in college work is more important than the subjects that have been pursued." Interestingly, Lowell followed up his remarks with a comment specifically about the need for courses in chemistry as an undergraduate. Contradicting the principal premedical focus on the study of chemistry that had been established by his predecessor, Charles W. Eliot (a chemist), Lowell suggests, "No doubt a certain command of chemistry, for example, is necessary. . . . But this may be acquired in ways other than college courses."[41]

Despite Lowell's suggestion, an important change took place in 1914 in Harvard's admission requirements for its medical school. For the first time two years of undergraduate chemistry were required: one year in inorganic chemistry and one year in organic chemistry. Michigan had switched in 1913 from one year of required chemistry to two years. Columbia switched to two years of chemistry in 1916; the University of California switched in 1915. Consistent with the state-mandated adherence to the admission requirements established by the AAMC, Stanford first required both inorganic chemistry and organic chemistry in 1919. Johns Hopkins had required two years of chemistry for some time.

By 1920, the established norm for premedical education had become a requirement of two years of chemistry, a year of physics, and a year of biology. This was the requirement at the six schools we have been following; it was becoming the national standard that was being enforced by a growing number of state licensing boards. Over a period of forty years, this series of required courses had evolved from the unorthodox to the orthodox. For the next seventy years this norm would change little. With the shift to English as the principal language for publication of medical research, the requirement of a reading knowledge of German and French has been dropped, as has any reference to a familiarity with Latin. More emphasis is placed on having taken undergraduate courses in English and mathematics. However, for a student applying to medical school in 1920, a student applying to medical school in 1951, and a student applying to medical school today, the requirements were the same: two years of chemistry, a year of physics, and a year of biology. As we will see in the following chapter, other than Lowell's study from 1911 that questioned these requirements, there was essentially no scientific evidence in 1920 that this mandated preparation in the sciences was a valid indicator of a student's "fitness to study medicine."

Questioning the Standard Premedical Curriculum, 1926–1952

At their annual meeting in 1925, the AAMC adopted a revised set of "minimum entrance requirements" that would be applied to its member schools. They published these requirements in 1926 in the inaugural issue of the *Bulletin of the Association of American Medical Colleges,* the association's new journal.[42] (Previously, the AAMC had relied on the *Journal of the American Medical Association,* and before that the *Bulletin of the American Academy of Medicine* to publish its proceedings.) Those requirements were largely the same as those of 1914. They called for 60 semester hours of collegiate instruction, with 30 hours comprising one academic year. Of the 60 hours spent as an undergraduate, 44 hours of specific classes were required, which included:

- Chemistry—16 hours
- Physics—10 hours
- Biology—12 hours
- English Literature and Composition—6 hours

While these 44 hours, comprising 73 percent of the available hours during the specified two years of college, were the minimum requirement, the AAMC also identified some additional classes that were "recommended" or "highly desirable." These additional, optional classes included: "a supplementary course in the elementary physical chemistry"; additional work in organic chemistry, including "a fair proportion of laboratory work"; and an elective course in physics "suitable for students who desire more knowledge of physics than the general course affords."

The AAMC listed no required or recommended course in French or German. By this time much of the then-current medical literature was published in English. As described by Dr. Hugh Cabot, dean of the University of Michigan Medical School, "The practice of the modern medical student does not use what knowledge he has [of French and German] and the time spent upon it may, therefore, be adjudged to have been largely wasted."[43]

To complete the subjects required by the AAMC in two years of college, a student would have to spend nearly all his time studying the premedical sciences. Even if a student spread his undergraduate work out over three years, he would be spending nearly two-thirds of his time in the science classroom or laboratory. Since these were the standards set by the AAMC, those states that had established their licensure laws based on those standards essentially forced premedical students to spend their college years focused almost exclusively on science. As more educators became aware of this issue, they began to voice concerns and reservations about the direction premedical education had taken.

Dean Hugh Cabot of Michigan voiced these concerns in the lead article in the inaugural issue of the AAMC's *Bulletin:*

> At the present time, the most striking characteristic of the premedical course is the large proportion of elementary science. . . . It seems not impossible that this large proportion of science as compared to what might be called "the Humanities" would be apt to result in the selection of students interested in science and having capacity in this field rather than those interested in the humanities and in mankind.
>
> I am not prepared to admit at the present time that in the equipment of the practitioner a knowledge of science is of more real value than a knowledge of the way in which mankind has behaved in the past and how he is on the whole behaving at the present time. The problems of medicine, on the whole, are quite as likely to require sound judgment based on a knowledge of history, sociology, philosophy and psychology as on the facts of science.[44]

Cabot is raising some of the same concerns Lowell raised in his cautions to the CME in 1914. These concerns were echoed in 1926 by Samuel P. Capen, the chancellor of the University of Buffalo. Capen suggested that "the transfer to the premedical curriculum of the basic sciences previously taught in medical school" had defeated the purpose initially established by the CME, that of assuring, "the broader and sounder general education of the physician." Capen asked, "Which is more important for the medical student, thorough grounding in the basic sciences or wider general education?"[45] Capen went on to suggest an experiment that, if carried out, would answer his question: the creation of an experimental, alternative curriculum, and a comparison of the quality of the premedical education in the experimental curriculum with that in the standard curriculum. His experiment "would set up for prospective physicians a curriculum . . . [that] would include a considerable amount of the social sciences, especially psychology, sociology, history, and economics. Necessarily the time allocated to scientific and linguistic preparation would be somewhat curtailed."[46]

A few months after the remarks of Drs. Cabot and Capen were published, Franklin D. Barker, a professor of zoology from Northwestern University, argued against any dilution of the premedical sciences. Speaking to the AAMC's national meeting held in October 1926, Prof. Barker described the practice at Northwestern: "In determining the fitness of the premedical student, we have applied the 'Harvard yardstick.' . . . In evaluating his scholarship, we have found that his record in the biological sciences was the most reliable index of his *fitness for the study of medicine* and his standing in chemistry the second best indicator" (emphasis added).[47]

This controversy over the extent to which science courses should predominate in the premedical curriculum raised concerns within the AAMC. In 1925 the AAMC appointed its own Commission on Medical Education (not to be confused with the AMA's Council on Medical Education). The commission was charged with conducting a study of the changing nature of medical education in the context of the changing needs of society. A. Lawrence Lowell, president of Harvard University, was appointed as chairman of the commission. Its secretary was Dr. Walter Bierring, representing the Federation of State Medical Boards of the United States. Hugh Cabot of Michigan and Samuel Capen of Buffalo were members of the commission, as was Dr. Ray Lyman Wilbur, president of Stanford University and formerly dean of the Stanford Medical School (1911–16), president of the AMA (1923–24), and president of the AAMC (1925–26). The individual chosen to conduct the actual study and to report on it was Dr. Willard C. Rappleye, then on the faculty of the Columbia College of Physicians and Surgeons, and from 1931–1958 the dean of that medical school. One of the first things the commission did was to negotiate with the Federation of State Medical Boards a moratorium on any new state-mandated premedical requirements until after the commission had completed its study and filed its report.

Dr. Rappleye published an article in 1930 describing the history and purpose of the commission. In his paper he paid particular attention to problematic issues that had arisen in premedical education: "Premedical subjects have been prescribed with little regard to the student's knowledge of these subjects. Many premedical subjects are subdivided into special fields of study which provide relatively little training in the most important features of the subject. . . . There seems to be little doubt but that a reorientation of the subject-matter in the preliminary sciences could easily provide students with a better comprehension of the principals of these subjects, not only for medicine but equally so for general education."[48]

The commission issued its final report in 1932.[49] The Report described its purpose as studying "the broader relationships of medical education to general and university education and to the shifting problems of medical practice, community health needs, and medical licensure" (2). The Report paid particular attention to the issue of premedical education. It identified the problems facing premedical education at that time: "The tendency of medical schools and regulatory bodies to define in detail the range and character of premedical preparation is contrary to the spirit of a real education, which should be general and not preprofessional in purpose. A sound general education is of more value to students of medicine than a narrow technical training in the premedical sciences" (267).

The authors of the Report acknowledged the growing practice among medical schools of using success in the premedical sciences to screen students for admission: "Inasmuch as most medical schools have a large number of applicants with more than the present minimum premedical education than they can accept, there is little inclination to change their policy of giving preference to the applicants who . . . present the best preparation. . . . The increase in premedical education has been due in part to the desire of medical school officers to set up mechanical or objective methods of selecting students" (270–71). The authors expressed concern over this mechanistic approach. As they saw it, "It is not wise to create detailed requirements which make it difficult for superior students who may not have followed a prescribed course of earlier education to study medicine" (271). Rather, the authors recommended that medical schools recognize "that the most important requirements for admission to medicine are character, ability, personality, a mind prepared by a sound plan of general education, and a grasp of the principles upon which medicine is dependent" (272).

As described in the commission's Report, part of the problem in creating a premedical curriculum that over-emphasizes the sciences is the tendency of science instructors to teach not just the principles of their discipline, but a level of detailed knowledge that is only useful to practitioners within that science:

Much of the science teaching is presented from the special interest of the teacher or the department. Organic chemistry is frequently taught from the standpoint of the dyes and similar industrial uses and much or inorganic chemistry emphasizes its commercial applications. . . . Physics is likely to be taught in its relationships to engineering and industry. . . . In general these subjects are not presented from the point of view of either general education or the specific preparation for medicine, but from that of preparation for advanced work in the separate sciences. (274)

The authors of the Report state their conclusions regarding premedical education in very explicit terms:

There has been a tendency on the part of individual medical schools to increase the premedical requirements, particularly in chemistry. . . . It is quite likely that the medical profession is losing men and women of high native ability and character who desire to study medicine and who have not been able to meet the specific premedical requirements in the usual college course. . . .

An adequate knowledge of the principles and methods of these sciences for the purposes of medical education could probably be secured more satisfactorily by good students in less time than is now required . . . if the course were modified and focused properly upon the needs of the student. A change in the methods of presentation and in the motivation of the present courses, rather than additions, is needed. (275)

The authors offer a clear message to the admissions committees of medical schools: "It is probably true that a considerable number of very well qualified and desirable students are lost to medicine each year through the insistence on the letter rather than the spirit of the regulations regarding premedical education. The character, personality, ability, and promise of the student rather than specific courses and credit hours in prescribed subjects are the important factors to be considered" (277–78).

In closing the section of the Report that focused on premedical education, the authors state:

A sound general training is of more value as preparation for the study of medicine than a narrow, technical training limited largely to the premedical sciences. . . . Attention in the selection of students should be given to evidence of a grasp of the principles and philosophy of the scientific method, rather than to the amount and division of time spent in individual subjects. . . .

It is a question of different, not longer or more courses in physics, chemistry, and biology and of discrimination in the subject matter and illustrative laboratory exercises. (282)

Less than two decades after the CME and the AAMC had called for more strict enforcement of premedical standards by medical schools and state licensing boards, leaders of those same organizations were calling for restraint. It seems that as an unintended consequence of their efforts to standardize premedical education around a series of courses in chemistry, biology, and physics, the quality of the general education of college students hoping to become physicians had been impaired. These leaders called on medical schools to de-emphasize premedical sciences and broaden the criteria by which they selected medical students.

It is one thing to admonish medical schools to de-emphasize the sciences in their admission process, but it is altogether another to actually see that change come about. Speaking to the Premedical Club of Amherst College in 1936, Dr. Harold Plough, professor of biology at Amherst, cautioned premedical students at Amherst about what it took to get into medical school. He read to them an excerpt from the final report of the Commission on Medical Education. He then acknowledged for his audience the reality of medical school admissions in 1936: "In spite of all the statements that training in a non-specific field is desirable, *the schools continue to show preference for those whose advanced training has been in one of the fundamental scientific fields*" (emphasis added).[50] For premedical students at Amherst in the 1930s, it was best to have as the "purpose of life" success in chemistry, biology, and physics—despite what the authors of the CME's Report said.

Encouraging a Liberal Education versus Using Science Classes to "Weed out" Students

The years surrounding World War II saw a series of changes in medical education and premedical education made to accommodate the war effort and the surge in the need for medical personnel associated with the war. After the war things settled down somewhat, but a growing tension developed between the need to encourage and support a broad liberal education among premedical students and the tendency to select students for medical school based on their performance in chemistry, biology, and physics. Increasing national emphasis was being placed on using standardized tests, combined with grades in the premedical science classes, to select students for medical school.

Writing in 1948, F. J. Mullen, dean of students at the University of Chicago Medical School, cited the worrisome statistics that 11 percent of the approximately 6,000 students who entered medical school in 1946 were no longer enrolled after the first year. For the class that entered medical school in 1944, 15 percent failed to graduate. "If we could so select our students as to eliminate at the start this 15 percent who are apparently intellectually or emotionally unable to make the grade," Mullen suggested, "we could increase the output of trained physicians from our schools by this quantity without the necessity of starting any new schools or spending any more money than we do now for medical education."[51] Mullen described research being done at his medical school to use a combination of undergraduate grades and the results of various personality tests to select the best students for medical school.

Writing in that same year, Donald B. Tressider, president of Stanford University, cautioned about the negative aspects of relying too heavily on students' performance in the premedical sciences, suggesting, "We require, therefore, an exhaustive re-examination of both medical and premedical education." Tressider identified what he saw as two fundamental weaknesses of the American system of medical and premedical education: "First, many of our graduates are, indeed, well trained technically but are poorly educated. Not only have we failed to provide them with a broad, general education, but all too many of them are deficient in the primary art of communication. . . . Secondly, many of our graduates do not possess an adequate understanding of the social problems of our complex modern society and fail to realize the extent of their own social responsibility." Tressider described the untoward effects of a premedical curriculum that is too heavily structured around the sciences: "By our insistence on strict adherence to definite patterns of courses at the college level as a condition of admission to medical school . . . we have contributed significantly to the growing chaos in general education." He closed his paper by saying, "As medical educators, we must be concerned with education at all levels and lose no opportunity to participate in the broad purposes of our entire education system to the end that we produce competent doctors who are above all else responsible citizens."[52] (Shortly after Tressider made these remarks, he died suddenly while on a trip to New York.)

Responding to the continuing concerns about the potential adverse effects of an overly structured premedical curriculum, in 1947 the AAMC and the CME appointed a joint committee to undertake a Survey of Medical Education. A core element of this survey was to be the Subcommittee on Preprofessional Education, to be chaired by Dr. Aura Severinghaus, dean of admissions at the Columbia College of Physicians and Surgeons. The subcommittee gathered data from 115 undergraduate colleges and universities, seeking to address three issues: (1) to define the qualifications that a person should have for a successful career in medicine, (2) to ascertain the extent to which undergraduate colleges are producing the kind of students the medical schools need, and (3) to make certain recommendations on the basis of their investigation.[53] The subcommittee issued its report in 1953, corroborating many of the concerns expressed by Dr. Rappleye and the Commission on Medical Education in 1932 and President Tressider in 1948:

Unfortunately, however, the medical profession and the present medical school admission requirements are attracting to our liberal arts colleges, as the gateways to medical school, a vocationally oriented group of students, many of whom have little interest in those items typically in the undergraduate program which, in their opinion, do not obviously contribute quite directly to the occupational objectives. . . . These students have little or no conception of the meaning of a liberal education; they have come to college to prepare themselves to earn a living.[54]

On the very next pages, however, the authors begin to discuss the flip side of the issue of premedical education: assuring that students who enter college with the intention of studying medicine are indeed fit to study medicine:

The liberal arts college, therefore, has the important responsibility of trying to prevent students from cherishing inappropriate professional ambitions too long. . . . Effort should be made as early in the student's college career as possible to determine whether, on the basis of personality, character, motivation, and academic performance, he is qualified to go into medicine. If it is decided he is not qualified, then every intelligent device, including aptitude and interest tests, should be used to persuade him to reevaluate his professional objective.[55]

The authors seem to be arguing simultaneously that (a) it is important for colleges to encourage premedical students not to sacrifice the quality of their general education by taking too many science courses; and (b) it is the college's responsibility to identify students who are not "qualified to go into medicine" and to "persuade them to reevaluate" their professional aspirations.

The authors of the report go on to make a statement that holds particular relevance in light of the comments of the students in our research study described in chapter 1. Once students who do not perform well in the early premedical sciences are "persuaded" to reevaluate their career goals, the authors then ask about "the extent of the responsibility which the undergraduate college should assume for those students who are *weeded out* of the group seeking admission to medical school"[56] (emphasis added). The authors were clear on the form this "weeding out" process takes at many schools: "We noted also an unduly tough attitude on the part of many chemistry teachers who claim with pride that only students of good ability who work very hard can get through their chemistry course."[57]

By the 1950s, medical schools had acknowledged a fundamental need to reduce the number of students who were selected for medical school but who, for either personal or academic reasons, were unable to complete medical school. The way they approached this issue was to identify explicit predictors of medical school fail-

ure and then to identify those premedical students who exhibited these characteristics. While sometimes the characteristics used to "weed out" students were personality traits, most often it was a student's early performance in science courses,
principally chemistry, that was used to this end. In 1893, Daniel Coit Gilman had
described the use of the premedical curriculum established at Johns Hopkins in 1878
to "prune and graft our promising vines."[58] In 1953, Aura Severinghaus described
how that same curriculum should be used to "weed out" students who are not "qualified to go into medicine." One of the Stanford students quoted in chapter 1 seems
to be describing precisely this process when he described Stanford's premedical curriculum and the adverse impact it had had on his aspirations for becoming a physician: *"Everyone says it's more like a weeding-out process than anything [else] and I just
ended up being one of those people."*

The 1953 Subcommittee Report commented on the growing pressure experienced by premedical students. They acknowledged that "students who get poor
grades in the sciences and rely on better grades in the nonscience courses frequently
have trouble getting into medical school."[59] This pressure to get high grades in the
science courses had led to a growing sense of competition among premedical students, resulting in precisely the type of outcome the subcommittee had hoped colleges would avoid: "Although the situation is much improved today, many medical
schools in the past have used achievement in the physical and biological sciences,
measured in terms of academic grades, as their principal yardstick in evaluating applicants for admission. Acting on the impression that this practice still prevails, the
premedical student devotes himself assiduously to these subjects, sometimes to the
neglect of the nonscience part of his program."[60]

Commenting on the effects of these perceptions on the culture of premedical education, Daniel Funkenstein of the Department of Psychiatry of Harvard Medical
School wrote in 1955 about the plight faced by the premedical student: "Seeking council from his colleagues, premedical advisors, doctors, and friends, he becomes more and
more anxiety ridden as he contemplates the almost super-human test before him of securing entrance to medical school. With great trepidation he . . . enters what the Harvard Crimson calls the 'rat race.'" Funkenstein cautioned that "when medical schools
state, as they have in recent publications, their opposition to such educational practices,
and their belief in a broad liberal education as the best preparation for medical school,
they are met with a very resistant attitude."[61] It is all well and good for medical schools
to preach the benefits of a broad liberal education. The premedical students knew,
however, at least in the 1950s, that the true orthodoxy of medical school admissions expected from the students success in chemistry, biology, and physics.

In 1957 the AAMC held a special Teaching Institute to follow up on these issues.

In its report, *The Appraisal of Applicants to Medical Schools,* the AAMC again acknowledged the importance of balancing intellectual characteristics (such as grades in chemistry) and nonintellectual characteristics (such as motivation, emotion, and integrity) in selecting students for medical school.[62] While we will consider in the following chapters the specific methods they proposed for measuring and assessing these characteristics, the comments of one workshop participant are especially pertinent. T. R. McConnell, professor of education and director of the Research Project in Higher Education at the University of California, Berkeley, pointed out that "in the case of medicine . . . we have the problem of predicting at least two things: first, success in medical school, and second, professional performance."[63] From the time studies of predictors of medical school performance first began in the 1930s to the period of the 1950s, predicting "success" in medical school meant either predicting who would graduate from medical school and who would not, or who would get high grades in medical school and who would not. McConnell was pointing out that an equally important outcome to measure was how good a physician a student would eventually become.

Those attending the conference agreed that there were several measures available (of varying validity and reliability) to predict performance in medical school but almost no valid means of predicting quality as a practicing physician. This point was emphasized by Funkenstein, who said, "The importance of research in this area cannot be emphasized too much. We need follow-up studies beyond medical school of both the men accepted and those rejected. The most pressing, and in many ways the most difficult item on such a research agenda would be successful criteria of a successful medical career."[64]

For a period of decades following the studies published in the 1950s by the AAMC, discussion and debate would continue surrounding the issues of obtaining a broad liberal education vs. preparation in the sciences and of selecting students based on performance in the sciences vs. using noncognitive predictors of ultimate quality as a physician. In 1961 the Commonwealth Fund published a book edited by Dr. George Miller of the University of Illinois College of Medicine in which he and his fellow authors wrote of the "thankless task" faced by medical school admissions committees "to discriminate from a pool of applicants the potentially good medical student when the criteria by which the 'good medical student' can be identified have never been clearly delineated." Miller and his colleagues comment on the continuing dilemma facing the premedical student:

The problem is of the sort which sophisticated journalists like to refer to as schizophrenic. On the one hand, medical school catalogues and forceful spokesmen in the field of medical education exhort the student to gain breadth of vision, a sociological and humanistic orientation, a "liberal" education. On the other hand, admissions committees appear for the most part to emphasize academic, particularly scientific, achievement. The hopeful candidate's best bet is to follow what he perceives to be the policy of the admissions committee.

Miller closes with a comment about the medical school selection process: "But it must be kept in mind that the prediction concerns successful medical school performance, not successful performance as a physician. The latter awaits adequate demarcation of the characteristics of a good physician."[65]

In the 1970s, Lewis Thomas was one of the most respected writers in medicine, publishing a regular series of essays in the *New England Journal of Medicine* under the moniker Notes of a Biology Watcher. In May 1978, in one of these essays, titled "How to Fix the Premedical Curriculum," Thomas wrote, "The medical schools used to say they wanted applicants as broadly educated as possible, and they used to mean it. . . . There is still some talk in the medical deans' offices about the need for general culture, but nobody really believes it, and certainly the premedical students don't believe it. . . . They concentrate on science with a fury, and they live for grades."[66]

Thomas seemed to be describing precisely what Rappleye had described in 1930. In a series of papers published in 1999, historian Gert Breiger describes the evolution of the thinking about the balance between a broad liberal education and one focused on the sciences.[67] He points out that while medical schools have historically emphasized the sciences, they have come to realize that majoring in science as an undergraduate gives little advantage to a student compared to selecting a major in a non-science subject. Studies by Dickman and colleagues[68] and by Zeleznik and colleagues[69] confirm Breiger's assessment.

A review of the admissions policies of the medical schools we have been following confirms Breiger's view that by the 1960s a student's choice of a major had little effect on his chances of admission, at least in theory. As early as 1960, the bulletin of the Harvard Medical School stated, "Provided [the applicant] is able to demonstrate competence in the natural sciences, the field of his college major will not influence consideration of him by the Admission Committee." In 1981 the bulletin of the medical school at the University of California, San Francisco, stated that, in addition to the science and math prerequisites, "Humanities courses such as literature, history, and the arts are recommended to provide the best basis for increasing students' understanding of human beings." In 2000, the Columbia bulletin stated, "The student may have concentrated on any subject—in the natural sciences, social sciences, humanities, or arts—but evidence of a balanced education, as well as demonstrated interest and ability in the natural sciences, is preferred." Despite these clear statements that premedical students should feel free to select the undergraduate major that interests them most, a study of medical students entering the UCLA School of Medicine in the early 1990s found that "the overwhelming majority of our medical students still major in the natural sciences during their college years, despite an admissions policy that allows for the acceptance of students with a broad range of academic backgrounds."[70]

It may be accurate to say that today an English major can stand on an equal footing with a biology major in the eyes of most medical school admissions committees, provided that student has performed well in the required courses in chemistry, biology, and physics. However, it is still true, as we observed in chapter 1, that at both Stanford University and the University of California, Berkeley, incoming freshmen who aspire to become physicians face substantial pressure to enter the established premedical curriculum early in their college careers. In most cases this means enrolling in freshman chemistry, followed in sequence by courses in biology and physics.

The expectation of undergraduate courses beginning with chemistry early in the college experience, followed by courses in physics and biology, became the norm for medical school admissions between 1893 and 1905 because people like Daniel Coit Gilman, M. Carey Thomas, Charles W. Eliot, and Victor C. Vaughan believed fervently that these courses, modeled on the German model of medical education, were an absolute prerequisite for any student to attain the status of "Fit to Study Medicine," as Gilman referred to it. Their belief was an essential part of their wider belief that only by infusing medical education with a core of scientific knowledge could medical practice in the United States become part of the modern era. But their belief was just that—a belief. They neither had, nor felt the need to have, scientific data to support their belief that only through college courses in chemistry, biology, and physics could a student be adequately prepared for medical school. Because they believed it, they worked (very effectively) to make that belief the standard of premedical education for the twentieth century.

Today English majors can go to medical school, so long as they do well in chemistry, biology, and physics. Economics majors can go to medical school, so long as they do well in chemistry, biology, and physics. Art majors can go to medical school, so long as they do well in chemistry, biology, and physics. The earlier they start their chemistry, the more competitive they will be when they enter the medical school admissions process. This is the mantra students at Stanford and UC Berkeley hear when they enter college. I suspect it is the mantra most college freshmen who aspire to become physicians hear as soon as they walk on the college campus.

In 1893 Daniel Coit Gilman used the metaphor of pruning a vine to describe the need to select for medical school only those students with an adequate preparation in the undergraduate sciences. In 1980 Dr. Edmund Pellegrino published an editorial in *JAMA* that used the metaphor in a different way. In his article Pellegrino criticized the historical tendency of medical school admissions committees to "[make] their choices on the strength of the Medical College Admissions Test scores in science or in that eternal verity—organic chemistry." For most members of medical school admissions committees, "the idea that medicine is synonymous with science is so inextricably insinuated into their minds that it is now an ideology." Pellegrino acknowledged the difficulty in changing deeply rooted ideas: "If there is anything harder than planting a new idea, it is uprooting an old one. Everyone shrinks from the periodic pruning that old ideas demand if they are to remain healthy. To evict an old idea is to precipitate a panic of identity."[71]

In 2007 I attended a national meeting that addressed the need to increase the racial and ethnic diversity of the health professions in the United States. At that conference we heard from a panel of three health professionals—one physician, one nurse, one medical student—all from underrepresented racial or ethnic groups. Each had been remarkably successful; each had experienced severe difficulty in early undergraduate science courses. During a coffee break after their presentation as I was chatting with the head of a leading university, I remarked, "The panelists we just heard from certainly don't fit the model. Maybe the model is broken." The university leader replied, "No it's not. Everyone needs two years of chemistry, a year of biology, and a year of physics before they can go to medical school." Without thinking much about it, and adopting my best social-scientific skepticism, I asked him, "Can you prove that?"

Much to my embarrassment, he became quite angry, refusing to discuss the matter further and gesticulating as he turned and walked away. I had not meant to be flip or disrespectful. I had genuinely wanted to know if he had ever considered whether his obviously deeply rooted belief in the role of chemistry, biology, and physics was supported by scientific data.

Pellegrino's editorial had been in response to the article by Dickman and colleagues, cited above. That article concluded that "one's undergraduate major does not lead to an appreciable difference in subsequent performance in the clinical sciences of medical school."[72] As Pellegrino suggested in his editorial, "These conclusions will be heretical to many educators."[73] My discussion with the university leader was not about a student's choice of major. It was about the expectation that all premedical students must have courses in chemistry, biology, and physics. It appears that to him my remarks were heretical.

In 1997, *Academic Medicine,* the journal of the AAMC, published an exchange of letters that addressed this apparently controversial issue. Dr. Pascal Imperato of State University of New York, Brooklyn, suggested that the "trend in medical education should logically lead to a discussion about reforming premedical undergraduate requirements in biology, general and organic chemistry, mathematics, and physics. Yet such a discussion has hardly begun."[74] Members of a working group established by the AAMC responded to Dr. Imperato's suggestion: "First, the working group believes that medicine must continue to be a science-based profession, and therefore undergraduate requirements in chemistry, general and inorganic chemistry, and physics are essential."[75]

Recall the comments of Dr. Ezekiel Emanuel in JAMA in 2006, cited in chapter 1. Dr. Emanuel asked, "Why are calculus, organic chemistry, and physics still premed requirements? Mainly to 'weed out' students. Surely, it would be better to require challenging courses on topics germane to medical practice, research, or administration to assess the quality of prospective medical students, rather than irrelevant material."[76] As did Dr. Imperato's suggestion in 1997, Dr. Emanuel's suggestion that we prune the historical premedical requirements met with strident opposition.

The controversy continues. Are courses in chemistry, biology, and physics essential to premedical education? Would a reformed premedical curriculum adversely affect the quality of the medical practice of the graduates of such a reformed curriculum? These questions await an answer derived from well-designed scientific observation. While we wait, substantial numbers of highly qualified college students at places such as Stanford and UC Berkeley, many of them from underrepresented racial and ethnic groups, enter the chemistry classroom in the belief that becoming a physician requires them to be there, only to have their professional aspirations founder. In the following chapters, in an effort to address these questions, I review the data that allows us to identify which factors accurately predict success in medical school and in medical practice.

CHAPTER FOUR

Premedical Education and the Prediction of Professional Performance

In the case of medicine . . . we have the problem of predicting at least two things: first, success in medical school, and second, professional performance.

T. R. McConnell, 1957

By 1920 premedical education had become largely standardized in the United States. Medical schools differed somewhat on the expected length of the premedical education—some expected only two years of college, while some required a bachelor's degree. However, nearly all medical schools required college courses in chemistry, biology, and physics. Once a student had successfully passed these courses, he was then eligible for admission.

The creation of this national norm for premedical education was not based on scientific evidence linking it with a higher standard of professional practice for the new graduates. Rather, it was grounded in the widely held belief that medical education must by its very nature be based in science—both education in medical school and premedical education in colleges and universities. This was the model of medical education the United States had imported from Europe starting in the late 1800s.

As long as there was a place in medical school available to every undergraduate who had successfully completed the required sequence of premedical courses, the level of a student's performance in those courses, either his absolute level or his level relative to his premedical peers, seemed less important. This was to change, however, beginning in mid-1920s, when for the first time the number of applicants to medical schools nationwide was greater than the number of the available places in medical schools.

Recall from the previous chapter that, largely as a result of the efforts of the American Medical Association (AMA), the Association of American Medical Colleges (AAMC), and a series of laws regulating medical practice passed in a number of states, the number of medical schools in the United States decreased from more than 160 in 1910 (the year the Flexner Report was published) to 85 in 1920. Coincident with the rising professional status of the medical profession during this era, an increasing number of college students became interested in a medical career. Between 1926 and 1935 the number of applicants to medical school nationwide increased by 50 percent.[1] Between 1926 and 1927 alone, applicants increased by 32 percent.[2] The combination of a decrease in the number of medical school slots, accompanied by an increase in the number of medical school applicants, inevitably led to the need to develop mechanisms to select from among those applying for admission those students who were the most "fit to study medicine."

The problems this situation presented were discussed in a paper presented to the annual meeting of the AAMC in 1926 by Dr. John Wyckoff of the New York University Medical College. In 1919 NYU had experienced for the first time a greater number of applicants than available slots. Beginning in 1921, NYU had created its first Admissions Committee, charged with selecting among these applicants. In describing the admissions criteria used by the committee, Wyckoff stated: "Obviously, three requirements are fundamental: mental equipment, physical equipment, and that quality so difficult to define—character. While it is undoubtedly true that a poor or mediocre student, if he has the usual character, will make a better physician than a man of high scholarship with less character, still, there is a minimum of mental ability that is essential if he is to carry the medical curriculum."[3]

By "carry the medical curriculum," Dr. Wyckoff means not to fail the first years of medical school. Between 1910 and 1920, the number of NYU medical students who failed the first year of medical school ranged between 20 and 40 percent. Dr Wyckoff commented that "the usual wastage, which comes from a large percentages of failures at the end of the first and second year, is partly unnecessary and should be avoided."[4] To avoid this "wastage," NYU began to look for an association between a student's grades in the first year of medical school and his grades in the premedical sciences. The association was clear: the group of students with the highest premedical grades also had the highest medical school grades; those with the lowest premedical grades had the lowest medical school grades. Beginning in 1922, they used this association to select students for admission, accepting those students with the best grades in the premedical sciences. Within a few years the failure rate at the end of the freshman year had been cut to less than 6 percent. Commenting on the success of this new program, Dr. Wyckoff remarked, "It is interesting to see how the wastage at the end of the first year at medical school may be cut by giving heed to the collegiate standing of students."[5]

In 1928 Dr. Frederick van Beuren reported similar data from Columbia's medical school, coming to a somewhat different conclusion. While Wyckoff had looked only at undergraduate grades in the premedical sciences, van Beuren looked both at grades in the sciences and overall undergraduate grades. "We found, to our surprise, that the average grade of all the subjects studied was a better indication of character of the work of a student would do in the medical school than the average grade of the premedical required subjects alone."[6]

Before Wyckoff and van Beuren presented their data, there had been few published studies of factors that predict success in medical school. A literature review conducted by the American Council on Education and reported in 1929 of 3,650 reports of educational research published in the preceding ten years "found only seven related to medical education."[7] One of these seven, however, is of substantial importance and presents a somewhat different conclusion from Wyckoff's study.

At the 1914 meeting of the AMA's Council on Medical Education (CME), A. Lawrence Lowell, who had become president of Harvard University in 1909, cautioned delegates against adopting an overly rigid premedical education based primarily in the sciences, suggesting that such a curriculum "may have the effect of excluding able men from the profession."[8] Lowell cited research he had published in 1911 on the success of Harvard medical students.[9] Looking at the undergraduate and medical school experiences of students who had attended both Harvard College and Harvard Medical School between 1895 and 1910, Lowell asked whether a student's undergraduate performance in the sciences or his overall performance in his undergraduate studies was the better predictor of medial school success. Rather than using Wyckoff's measure of success (first-year medical school grades), Lowell looked to see which students had graduated from medical school with cum laude honors distinction. The highest rate of honors distinction was among students who had focused their undergraduate studies in literature, languages, philosophy, or mathematics, leading Lowell to conclude "that natural science in college is certainly not a markedly better preparation for the study of medicine than other subjects."[10] Lowell acknowledged that "the young man who has acquired some familiarity with natural science and the use of instruments has, no doubt, an initial advantage in the study of medicine, and is much easier to teach at the outset" [i.e., the first year of medical school] . . . but that . . . initial advantage was soon overcome in the course of professional study." Thus, as far as Lowell was concerned, "one subject is not distinctly better than another as a preparation for professional education."[11]

The quote at the beginning of this chapter by T. R. McConnell, founder of the Center for Studies in Higher Education at the University of California, Berkeley, sets out an important underlying issue in studies of the factors that predict or are associated with professional success. There are two ways of measuring success: academic success, and professional success. Grades in the first year of medical school represent a form of academic success; being recognized for distinction in overall medical school performance, pre-clinical as well as clinical, is a more general form of professional success. As we will see below, for much of the twentieth century, medical school admissions committees were concerned principally with predicting early academic success in medical school. It was only in the second half of the century that educators began to look more seriously at measures of professional success as indicated by the level of clinical skills of a practicing physician.

Predicting Early Academic Success in Medical School with Standardized Exams

By 1928 most medical schools were facing the problem of high rates of early failure among medical students. As described by Burton Myers, dean of the medical school at Indiana University, "The enrollment of 120 freshmen with the expectation of having 100 sophomores the following year, dropping 20 students whose year has cost an average of $700.00 per student, a loss of $14,000.00, is not economically justifiable if we can get our 100 sophomores by a more discriminating selection of 110 or fewer freshmen at a saving of $7,000.00 or more of school budget, the salary of a full-time staff man."[12] In speculating about how medical schools might avoid this "wastage," as Wyckoff had referred to it, Myers cited a study from the educational psychology literature published in 1923 in which Mark May of Syracuse University had used the results of two separate intelligence tests given to 450 incoming college students to predict their grades in college. Myers concluded that "the most reliable means of predicting academic success is a combination of intelligence and degree of application [i.e., effort]."[13]

In 1923 the use of intelligence tests was fairly new. One of the first was developed in 1905 by French psychologist Alfred Binet and was used to identify young children who were likely to have trouble in school due to their sub-par intelligence. Binet was later to collaborate with Lewis Terman at Stanford University to define the concept of intelligence quotient, or IQ, as the ratio of a subject's mental age (as measured on the new intelligence test) to the subject's physical age. As described by Nicholas Leman, in the years leading up to World War I, Terman and others "were tireless advocates of the widest possible use of IQ testing by American educators, so that students could be assessed, sorted, and taught in accordance with their capabilities."[14]

In the early use of the concept of IQ, intelligence was seen as an inherent human trait, something with which one is born. Intelligence tests could be used to identify slow learners who needed extra help in school, and it could be used to identify those with the potential for higher education. "The idea of IQ testers was not to reform education, especially higher education, so much as to reserve it for highly intelligent people, as indicated by IQ scores, lest their talents be wasted."[15]

When World War I came in 1914, the U.S. Army arranged for Prof. Robert Yerkes of Harvard to administer an IQ test to nearly two million recently recruited soldiers in order to identify those recruits best suited for training as officers. The success of IQ testing in this regard substantially increased both the general awareness of and the belief in intelligence testing as a valuable educational tool.

Evaluating the intelligence of physicians in the army during World War I yielded some interesting results. It turns out that Medical Officers in the army scored consistently lower on the battery of intelligence tests than did officers in the Engineer or Field Artillery Corps.[16] Further sub-set analysis showed the measured intelligence of Medical Officers varied substantially according to the AMA classification of the medical school from which they graduated: those graduating from schools ranked as "Class A" scored the highest on the army's intelligence test, while those graduating from schools ranked as "Class C" scored the lowest. It is also interesting to note that graduates of homeopathic schools of medicine scored substantially higher than even the graduates of "Class A" "regular" schools.

Carl Campbell Brigham was a psychology professor at Princeton. Working to adapt the intelligence test used by the army during World War I for use in a broader educational context, Brigham used a combination of mathematical calculations, identification of facial expressions, and word recognition to create a new test to use in the assessment of the intelligence of would-be college students: the Scholastic Aptitude Test, or SAT. The SAT, later to become the national standard in assessing the academic qualifications of high school students, was administered for the first time in 1926 to 8,040 high school students who were applying to college.

The American Council on Education (ACE) is an organization that represents colleges and universities. In 1929 its assistant director, David Allan Robertson, addressed the AMA's Annual Congress on Medical Education. Robertson described the work of Dr. F.A. Moss of George Washington University Medical School in adapting the SAT for use in evaluating applicants to medical school.[17] Moss's "scholastic aptitude test for medical school" was both a test of general intelligence and a test of one's knowledge of the premedical sciences. It included six sections:

1. a test of scientific vocabulary
2. a test of premedical information
3. a visual memory test based on having viewed for ten minutes a diagram of the heart and the major blood vessels

4. a verbal memory test based on having read a paragraph about the heart and the major blood vessels
5. a reading comprehension test
6. a test described as "understanding of printed material"

Moss had administered this test to the 1927 freshman medical school class at George Washington and, based on the test results, predicted which students would fail in medical school and which would attain academic distinction. Eight of the ten students predicted to fail did so; six of the eight students predicted to attain distinction did so. Based on these results, the ACE printed large quantities of the new test and handed them out to delegates to the 1929 meeting to be used in assessing their current first-year students. Those who administered the tests could send them to Dr. Moss for scoring. Robertson noted that "Dr. Moss has undertaken to send the results to the deans in time for them to use the scores, if they so desire, in connection with the elimination of students at the close of the present year. Obviously, if convenient tests which will reliably predict academic success in professional schools can be worked out, a great waste can be avoided for the individuals and institutions which now are losing time and energy in trying to make educational adjustments which cannot be made."[18]

From the outset, the scholastic aptitude test for medical schools, later to become the MCAT, was used principally to weed out applicants who were predicted to fail the first year of medical school. By using the test to define and measure the level of scientific knowledge required to predict success in the first two years of medical school, Robertson suggested, it was then the job of the undergraduate institution, "to provide a curriculum more directly effective in training men and women for the medical profession and in helping to choose them wisely."[19]

Twenty-six medical schools administered the "medical aptitude test" (MAT) developed by Moss to their freshman medical school class, forwarding the tests to Moss for scoring and providing Moss with the students' first-year grades. Moss divided the approximately 900 students into deciles based on their test scores, and then sorted students grades into four categories: 90 or greater, 85–89, 75–79, less than 75 (described as "failure"). Presenting his results to the annual meeting of the AAMC held in 1929, he reported a clear association between MAT scores and first-year grades.[20] Of the students in the top decile, none failed, and 93 percent had grades of 80 or higher; of students in the bottom decile, 42 percent failed, and only 14 percent had grades of 80 or higher. The overall correlation between MAT score and grades was 0.59. This compared to a correlation between undergraduate grades in the premedical sciences and first-year medical school grades of 0.50.

While his results were impressive, Moss pointed out to the delegates a potential problem. While 42 percent of students in the bottom decile failed the first year of medical school, 58 percent passed all their courses, albeit with lower grades than many of their classmates. If, in an attempt to prevent the future failures from entering medical school, admissions committees had administered the MAT to these students as applicants and refused admission to all students scoring in the bottom 10 percent, a substantial number of students fully capable of passing the medical school curriculum would have been refused admission as well.

Moss developed what he referred to as a measure of the "efficiency" of an admissions screening criterion by comparing the percent of failures that would have been prevented by using a criterion to screen out applicants with the number of students in his sample attaining a grade of 85 or higher in their first year of medical school who would have been refused admission based on the device. He noted, "We secured the best results by combining the Aptitude Test scores with the premedical grades. When such a combined criterion was applied to the group on which records were available, we found that 94 percent of the failures would be eliminated, and 20 percent of those who would make 85 or above. . . . It is quite probable that the ideal method for selecting students will be a combination of this method with the results of the aptitude tests and the premedical grades."[21]

Moss proposed to the meeting that all schools in the AAMC begin to administer the MAT to applicants for admission and that they do it nationally on the same day. His office would take responsibility for scoring the tests and reporting the scores to the deans. Two motions were made to the delegates at the meeting: (1) "that the Association record its sense of the importance of the study of aptitude tests in relation to the acceptance of students in medical schools"; and (2) that "the Association appoint a committee to direct an experimental study of aptitude tests for admission to medical studies" in the manner suggested by Moss.[22] Both motions passed, apparently enthusiastically.

The newly established Special Committee on the Evaluation of the Aptitude Test for Medical Students took on the study of the MAT and how it should be used in the admissions process, reporting back to the AAMC on a regular basis. In 1935 the Special Committee reported on its research to date. Responding to Moss's concern that use of the test to eliminate potential failing students would also eliminate a substantial number of students who would pass their medical school courses, the committee suggested that "a common sense practical view of the problem would seem to be one in which it is admitted that the best criterion is the one which would eliminate the greatest number of failures and at the same time the fewest number of good students. . . . In a very real sense there is and can be, probably, no right or correct answer to the problem."[23] At a time when 20 percent of entering medical students had failed by the end of their first year, it is understandable that the AAMC and the deans of the medical schools were willing to refuse admission to otherwise capable students based on a low test score in order to reduce the number of failing students.

Not all those who read the committee's report agreed with this approach, however. Edward Thorndike, a leading educational psychologist from Teachers College at Columbia University, wrote the following comments: "Superficially, the tests look somewhat pedantic and over-specialized and over-weighted with memorizing; and they probably are better to predict success in the first two years of medical school than success later and throughout life. I imagine they are frankly designed to weed out the kind of persons who would be weeded out by the first two years of work in medical school."[24]

The committee reported additional data in 1938[25] and in 1940.[26] For the entering medical school class of 1936–37, 84 percent of all entering students had taken the MAT. Of students scoring in the lowest decile of test scores, 25 percent failed the first year of medical school (and of course, 75 percent passed the first year). Only 2 percent of students in the highest decile failed in the first year. In 1938–39, with 90 percent of entering medical students having taken the test, the failure rates were nearly identical: 22 percent of students in the bottom decile, and 3 percent in the top decile. Moss felt that he had convincing evidence that the MAT score, taken together with a student's grades in premedical sciences, provided the best tool for predicting which students would fail the first year of medical school.

Moss paid less attention to what happened to students after their first year or two of medical school. The issue of the clinical or professional skills ultimately developed by students seemed of little concern to him. In 1933 W. F. Kramer of the University of Chicago pointed out that "success in medical schools is best measured by the success of the graduates after they leave school."[27] This view was echoed by I. L. Kandel, professor of education at Teachers College of Columbia University. In a report commissioned by the Carnegie Foundation for the Advancement of Teaching (the original publisher of the Flexner Report), Kandel reviewed the use of aptitude tests in the admissions process of schools of medicine, law, and engineering, concluding that "aptitude tests can only discover whether a candidate is likely to succeed in the professional preparation selected. They do not indicate promise of future success in the practice of that profession."[28]

In the 1940 Special Committee report, Moss made an important observation: "We found that questions taken directly from the premedical sciences have a much higher selective value than do general cultural questions based on knowledge of art, music, drama, history, literature, etc., or questions based on geography and current events. . . . As a result of this study we have greatly increased the number of premedical information questions and practically eliminated questions of a more general type in constructing the new form of the test."[29] The MAT was becoming less a test of general scholastic aptitude and more a test of familiarity with the premedical sciences.

World War II and its aftermath brought a substantial increase in the number of students applying to medical school. Both the need to train doctors for the war and the entry of returning veterans into the educational system added even more pressure to those evaluating applicants for admission to medical school. Officials at the AAMC thought that Moss's MAT continued to have shortcomings in its ability to select among applicants most efficiently, so in 1946 they replaced it with a new test called the Professional Aptitude Test. In 1948 this test was renamed the Medical College Admission Test (MCAT), the name it has today. In a comparison of the MAT and the MCAT, R. B. Ralph and C. W. Taylor emphasized that, in the face of the rising number of applicants, "the task of selecting those best fitted for medical training and of eliminating misfits at the earliest possible moment becomes increasingly important."[30] Unfortunately, in comparing the power of the MCAT to that of the older MAT to predict grades in the first two years of medical school, Ralph and Taylor concluded that various parts of the new test "have zero or negligible value as predictors."[31]

Throughout the 1950s researchers continued to try to improve the process by which students were selected for medical school. By 1959 the MCAT had been modified and had four sub-sections: Verbal, Quantitative, Modern Society, and Science. A separate score was reported for each section. In a study of more than 12,000 students applying to the State University of New York College of Medicine in Brooklyn between 1950 and 1957, J. K. Hill found that the combined score of the science and quantitative sections had the strongest association with academic success in medical school, again measured as grades in the first year of school. The association between the Verbal Ability score on the MCAT and freshman success was substantially lower.[32]

Not everyone associated with medical school admissions was comfortable with the continuing emphasis on predicting success and avoiding failure in the first year of medical school. In a 1957 review of research on medical school admissions, Gottheil and Michael cautioned, "Presumably, the goal of medical education is to produce 'good' doctors of medicine. What constitutes the good doctor however, and how to evaluate the constituent factors remains the most perplexing problem in the field. . . . The use of medical school grades as a criterion against which to evaluate the success of a selection program is not only subject to criticism on the grounds that grades may not be correlated with the quality of later practice of medicine, but there is an even more basic idea to consider: whether medical school grades are in themselves statistically reliable." The authors went on to ask, "To what extent can or should a broad cultural background in the socio-humanistic field be sacrificed for outstanding achievement in science?"[33]

Broadening the Scope of the Admissions Assessment to Include Predictors of Clinical Performance

By the 1950s, a number of the leaders in medical education in the United States were becoming concerned with the overemphasis on using success in the premedical sciences to select students for medical school. To address this issue, the AAMC convened a four-day teaching institute in 1956 at which representatives from most U.S. medical schools met to discuss "The Appraisal of Applicants to Medical School." The conference was to address the following question: "Is medicine attracting those students who are best endowed with the characteristics most favorable for serving the health needs of society and the research needs of medical science?"[34]

In addressing this question, the AAMC first administered a survey to administrators and admissions committee members at 91 medical schools in the United States and Canada. They then held a series of panel discussions and workshops to discuss the results of the survey. As reported by Dr. Robert Glaser, dean of the University of Colorado School of Medicine, the survey largely confirmed the heavy historic emphasis placed on performance in the premedical sciences, and on MCAT scores as a reflection of that performance.[35] Eighty-six percent of the schools reported placing great importance on science grades in evaluating applicants for admission, while 40 percent reported placing great emphasis on non-science grades. Fifty per cent of schools also placed great emphasis on MCAT scores. Among the premedical sciences, schools reported placing most emphasis on grades in the natural sciences, especially chemistry and physics, and only to a lesser degree biology. Similarly, schools reported giving most emphasis to an applicant's MCAT Science and Quantitative scores and relatively little emphasis to their Verbal Ability or Modern Society scores, leading Glaser to comment that "knowledge of modern society as measured by MCAT is not considered to be of major importance in the evaluation of the applicant's intellect."[36]

It was in response to statistics such as these that T. R. McConnell of the Center for Studies in Higher Education at the University of California, Berkeley, made his remark that leads off this chapter. What are we trying to do? McConnell asked. Are we trying to select those students who will do well academically in the early part of medical school, or are we trying to select those students who will make the best physicians after medical school? The two outcomes are not necessarily the same. This issue received substantial attention during the conference. Dael Wolfe, the executive officer of the American Association for the Advancement of Science, echoed McConnell's remarks. In trying to select the most qualified students, he said, "we must face the problem of deciding more highly qualified for what? More highly qualified in terms of what measures?"[37] R. F. Arragon, a professor of history from Reed College, concurred in the need to look beyond early success in the sciences, commenting that "there does seem to be some general assumption that there are qualities that may be necessary for success in the first two years—different qualities from those necessary for the clinical years to follow."[38] Commenting on the need to look beyond early medical school grades, Robert Glaser suggested, "Perhaps it is overly optimistic to suggest at this time that sound means of evaluating actual physician practice can be developed and that eventually selection measures may be validated against these more 'ultimate' criteria."[39]

The discussions at the conference of the need to broaden the perspective used in evaluating applicants to medical school were summarized by John Caughey, then associate dean at the Western Reserve School of Medicine:

> The principal result of the discussion of this topic was the realization by the participants of the great need for continuing well-organized study of medical student selection. . . . However the real challenge lies ahead and has not been accepted by medical faculties and admissions committees. This challenge is to define more precisely the expectations we have for members of the medical profession, to determine the intellectual and personal qualities which are necessary for the roles they are expected to play, and then to find means to attract, select, and educate the kind of students who, as physicians, will strive with reasonable hope of success to make the desired contributions to medical education, scientific research, and the health needs of their community.[40]

The AAMC conferees went on to discuss at some length the importance of including assessment of the nonintellectual characteristics of applicants as well as measures of their intellectual achievements, an issue I address in the chapter that follows.

The conference's emphasis on the pressing need to find ways to look beyond the first two years of medical school in gauging medical student success soon began to be reflected in the literature on premedical education. An important series of papers responding to this need began to appear in the early 1960s. In 1962 Schwartzman and colleagues from McGill University in Canada reported on their study of the association between the traditional markers of undergraduate performance and medical student grades in each of the four years of medical school. In looking at performance beyond the first year, they identified several important relationships:

- While there was an association between MCAT scores and student performance across all four years of medical school, the relationship was not as strong as had been previously reported of studies looking only at performance in the first year.
- There was an association between grades in the five required premedical subjects (the four sciences plus English) and student performance in the first year of medical school.
- By the fourth year there were no significant relationships between premedical grades and performance, although organic chemistry grades and English grades showed a weak association.[41]

In 1962 Funkenstein looked at which students leave before completing medical school. Rather than looking principally at who leaves after the first year, as most previous studies had done, he looked at students who left for any reason across all four years of medical school. He confirmed that the highest dropout rate was after the first year, with 5.5% of students leaving. The dropout rate decreased significantly after that: 2.1% after the second year, 1.1% after the third year, and 0.3% during the fourth year. Once students made it through the first year, nearly all were successful in completing medical school.[42] A later study by Gough and colleagues confirmed the substantially lower dropout rate after the first year, and indicated that those students who dropped out of medical school during the clinical years did so largely for personal rather than academic reasons.[43]

However, Funkenstein did notice a distinct pattern: those who dropped out during the first two years tended to be weaker in their premedical science and stronger in premedical humanities, while those who dropped out during the final two clinical years tended to be stronger in their premedical science and weaker in premedical humanities. A series of papers by Korman and colleagues supported the concept that, during medical school, students who were stronger in the undergraduate sciences than in the humanities tended to have different experiences and pursue different career goals than their colleagues who were stronger in the humanities.[44]

Richards and colleagues looked beyond medical school to assess the associations among premedical grades, MCAT scores, grades in medical school, and performance in the internship year immediately following medical school. The internship assessments reflected a global evaluation from the internship director of the intern's clinical skills. The authors concluded that "the best predictor of intern performance is grade average in the clinical year(s) of medical school, and that grades in the pre-clinical years of medical school [i.e., the first two years] have only a slight relationship to intern performance, and that premedical grades have almost no relationship."[45] Interestingly, the authors noted a negative but non-significant association between MCAT scores and intern performance, raising the possibility that the better a student did on the MCAT, the less well he or she did as an intern. Howell and Vincent also found a negative association between MCAT scores and evaluations of the clinical quality of interns.[46]

Johnson and colleagues took their evaluation one step further, looking at the association between medical school performance and clinical performance in a multi-year residency. They did not break down their assessment of medical school performance by year of school, but rather looked at a student's relative class standing across all four years. While students who ranked higher during medical school tended also to rank higher as residents, there was substantial crossover, with a number of lower-ranking medical students becoming high-ranking residents, and vice versa.[47]

Price and colleagues went beyond evaluations of postgraduate medical training to look at the professional skills of a sample of about 500 practicing physicians, representing academic practice, urban specialty practice, and both urban and rural general practice. They calculated a composite score of professional quality from a range of individual measures and then compared this score with premedical grades and medical school grades. The authors concluded, "Our study clearly demonstrates that performance in formal education, as measured by grade-point averages, comes out as a factor almost completely independent of all the factors having to do with performance as a physician."[48]

The *Journal of Medical Education* in which the Price and colleagues paper was published was the official journal of the AAMC. Following the Price article, the journal published the transcript of a discussion of Price's presentation of his results that had taken place at an AAMC meeting. That discussion posed a very interesting question, one that has continued relevance today. In response to the paper, Dr. George Saslow of the University of Oregon asked, "Suppose one of us had the power to start off a new medical school with a faculty willing to listen to data like this. In what directions would you suggest that we look in order to make predictions about the kinds of doctors that we need?" In response, Dr. Price replied: "The impression has grown on me more and more that since conventional grades and other measures used have been overweighted, difficult as it is, we are going to be forced to pay more attention to other qualities of character and personality, of behavior, of relationships to people, of matters of dedication and integrity. These things are hard to define and difficult to measure, but they may be the most important factors, and it may well be that they can be determined to some extent in medical students."[49]

Between 1963 and 1973, three separate groups of authors published comprehensive reviews of the literature linking academic performance and subsequent clinical skills.[50] Each supported the conclusion that the association between premedical performance and early medical school performance on the one hand with eventual clinical quality on the other was tenuous at best. Regarding faculty assessments of clinical quality in the fourth year of medical school, Gough and colleagues went so far as to suggest that "the MCAT scales and the three indices of premedical scholastic performance show an essentially zero relationship with this criterion."[51] Wingard and Williamson also found, "little or no correlation" between premedical grades and clinical performance.[52]

By the 1970s, medical schools had been using a combination premedical science grades and MCAT scores for more than forty years to select those students who were the most "fit to study medicine," as originally described by Daniel Coit Gilman in 1878. What if the criteria they had been using were not optimal? What if we could improve the overall clinical quality of the medical profession by using a different set of criteria to select from among the many applicants to medical school? If we could start from scratch, and given the growing body of research on the predictors of professional success in medicine, how would we structure our admissions process? Of course, we can't ignore history, nor can we expect members of medical school admissions committees simply to abandon processes that have evolved over a period of decades. However, the exchange between Drs. Saslow and Price raises intriguing questions.

Broadening the Effort to Predict Clinical Quality in the Selection of Medical Students

Research appearing in the 1980s and beyond and looking at factors associated with success in medical school typically included measures of clinical quality as well as academic quality. Clinical quality was often measured as performance in the clinical clerkships in the final two years of medical school and in the first postgraduate year of clinical training.[53] In one such study, DeVaul and colleagues took advantage of a natural experiment in which a public medical school was instructed by its state legislature to expand its entering class after the notices of acceptance and rejection had already been sent out. This unexpected expansion of medical school slots permitted the admissions office at the school to compare the medical school success of 50 students initially rejected but subsequently accepted with that of 150 students initially accepted. The authors concluded, "In attrition and in both pre-clinical and clinical performance through medical school and one year of postgraduate training, there were no meaningful differences between the groups."[54]

While there was general consensus on the need to include assessments of both academic performance and clinical quality, there was some concern that the measures used to assess clinical quality—typically the qualitative assessment of a clerkship director or internship director—did not provide as reliable a measure as did grades or standardized tests. Accordingly, researchers began to use a second measure of clinical quality in their research: scores on the national licensure examination administered by the National Board of Medical Examiners (NBME). Founded in 1915 as an independent nonprofit organization, NBME was charged with developing and administering a standardized licensure examination nationally. All medical graduates who wish to obtain a license to practice medicine must pass this exam. The exam was given in three parts: NBME I, testing knowledge of the preclinical sciences, given at the end of the second year of medical school; NBME II, testing clinical knowledge, given at the end of the fourth year of medical school; and NBME III, testing the application of clinical skills, given at the end of the first year of postgraduate studies (internship or residency). Using scores from these standardized examinations, researchers were able to have a more complete measure of success in medical school, to which they could compare measures of success in premedical studies, as illustrated in figure 4.1 below.

Using this general model of measuring outcomes of premedical and medical education, researchers were able to gain a more complete picture of those factors that predict success in medical school at the various stages of medical training. For example, in 1990 Dr. Karen Mitchell, vice-president for research at the AAMC and the director of the MCAT program, published her review of the literature linking premedical performance and medical school performance using this model. Using MCAT scores beginning in 1977, when the MCAT was reformulated to include more questions relating to scientific principles while eliminating questions pertaining to general knowledge of the liberal arts, Mitchell found that a combined measure of undergraduate GPA and MCAT scores was highly correlated with grades in the pre-clinical sciences ($r = 0.49$). Undergraduate performance had a weaker correlation with grades in the clinical years ($r = 0.38$) and with subjective assessments in the clinical years ($r = 0.27$). Similarly, undergraduate performance had the strongest correlation with the NBME I score ($r = 0.58$), less with the NBME II score ($r = 0.49$), and the weakest correlation with the NBME III score ($r = 0.35$).[55]

In 1993 Glaser and colleagues published their study addressing the following question: Among science, verbal, or quantitative skills, which is the best predictor

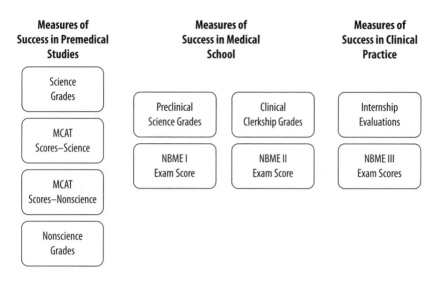

Figure 4.1. Measures of success in premedical studies and in medical school.

of physician competence? In a sample of 1628 graduates of Jefferson Medical College who had entered between 1978 and 1985, they used three MCAT scores as indicative of undergraduate performance: science problems, reading skills, and quantitative skills. They compared these measures with success in medical school as measured by parts I, II, and III of NBME and found that:

- Scores on the science problems subtest were better predictors of the basic science component of physician education (NBME I scores) than were the reading scores.
- Both science problems and reading skills predicted clinical science scores equally well (NBME II scores).
- Reading skills scores contributed more than the science problems subtest in predicting scores on an examination of patient management skills (NBME III scores).
- Scores on the quantitative skills subtest did not contribute to any prediction.[56]

From these results the authors concluded "that the verbal ability reflected in the reading skills scores of an applicant to medical school are more important indicators of later physician competence (as measured by standardized certifying examinations) than the applicant's ability to solve scientific problems."[57]

In a study of two graduating classes from a single medical school, Loftus and colleagues looked at predictors of performance in the first year of residency. They found that (1) subjective assessments of a student's performance in the clinical clerk-ships in medical school were the best predictor of performance in residency, and (2) undergraduate grades (science and non-science combined) had little relevance to performance in residency.[58]

Once researchers began to take a longer-term view of success in medical school, some clear patterns of associations began to emerge. In the era of approximately 1930–57, when researchers were concerned principally with preventing failure in the first year of medical school, it seemed both adequate and appropriate to use a stu-dent's performance in the premedical sciences, measured either as grades or science MCAT scores, to predict medical school success. However, when researchers began to expand their view of medical school success, they found that the factors that pre-dicted success in the first two years of medical school were only weak predictors of success in the final two years of medical school or of success in postgraduate train-ing (internship or residency). The factors that were linked most strongly with these later measures of professional success were skills in the humanities and general ver-bal skills.

In an effort to improve its predictive ability, the MCAT was revised in 1977 and again in 1991.[59] In order to balance the assessment of verbal ability and scientific knowledge, the 1991 version was divided into four parts: Biological Sciences, Physi-cal Sciences, Verbal Reasoning, and Writing Sample. Descriptions of the specific content areas for the four tests are available on the Web site of the AAMC.[60]

In 1996 research staff from both the AAMC and the NBME began to publish their studies of the new format for the MCAT and its ability to predict success in medical school. In one of the first studies, Swanson and colleagues looked spe-cifically at the accuracy of the new test in predicting the first step of the national licensing exam. (In 1992 the format of the NBME examination was changed some-what, and the name of the exam was changed to the United States Medical Licens-ing Examination [USMLE]; it was still developed and administered by the NBME and was administered in the same three steps as the previous NBME exam.) The au-thors described the purpose of the new MCAT as "to encourage students interested in medicine to pursue broad undergraduate study in the humanities and social sci-ences, as well as biology and the natural sciences. It emphasizes mastery of *basic* bi-ology, chemistry, and physics concepts; facility with scientific problem solving and critical thinking; and writing skills." In a study of 11,145 medical students, they found that the biological sciences and physical sciences components of new test were accurate predictors of USMLE I scores; that the verbal reasoning and writing sam-ple scores had little predictive ability of USMLE I scores; and that after taking into account scores on the biological sciences and physical sciences components of the

MCAT, neither undergraduate science grades nor undergraduate non-science grades added to the predictive accuracy of the MCAT scores alone.[61]

A study by Wiley and Koenig looked more carefully at the issue of the added value of premedical grades after taking into account MCAT scores. Taken alone, the correlation between grades and USMLE I scores (r = 0.43) was not as strong as the correlation between MCAT scores and USMLE I (r = 0.72). However, when grades and MCAT scores were taken together in a test of multiple correlations, the combination of the two measures added little to the association with the USMLE I scores (combined r = 0.75). When the authors looked at the association between premedical grades and MCAT scores with grades in the first two years of medical school, their results were essentially the same. This paper confirmed that MCAT scores alone are essentially as good at predicting USMLE I scores or grades in the first two year of medical school as is a combination of MCAT scores plus premedical grades.[62]

Dr. Ellen Julian, director of the MCAT for the AAMC, reported a follow-up study that she described as "a comprehensive summary of the relationships between [undergraduate] GPAs and MCAT scores and (1) medical school grades, (2) USMLE Step scores, and (3) academic distinction or difficulty." She noted a general pattern of decreasing rates of academic difficulty and increasing rates of academic distinction as MCAT scores increase. However she cautioned, "that incidents of distinction occur for students with very low MCAT scores, and incidents of difficulty occur for students with very high MCAT scores." Regarding the issue of the relative effects of MCAT scores and undergraduate grades (uGPAs) in predicting all aspects of medical school success, she concluded, "MCAT scores almost double the proportion of variance in medical school grades explained by uGPAs, and essentially replace the need for uGPAs in their impressive prediction of [USMLE] Step scores."[63]

Separating the MCAT into Its Constituent Parts

If MCAT scores seem to be the best predictor of success in medical school, the next question to address is whether the various sections of the test (biological sciences, physical sciences, verbal reasoning, writing sample) have similar or different associations with various levels of medical school success as measured by the three steps of the USMLE (scientific knowledge, clinical knowledge, clinical skills). Two recent research reports examined this question.

Veloski and colleagues looked at the records of several hundred medical students who entered Jefferson Medical College in the 1990s.[64] As measures of premedical

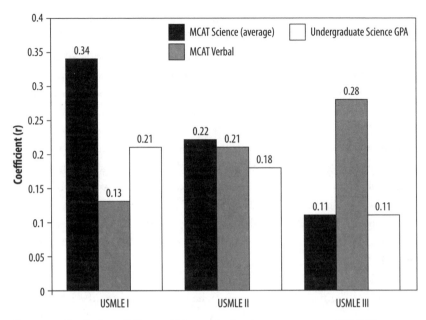

Figure 4.2. Predictive validity coefficients (r) of various measures on USMLE
Step Scores
Source: Data from Veloski et al., 2000

preparation they looked at students' undergraduate GPAs in their science courses
and their MCAT scores. For the MCAT scores they included the verbal reasoning
score and an average of the physical sciences and biological sciences scores. Using
multivariate analysis to take into account students' age, gender, and race/ethnicity,
the researchers looked at the correlations between these measures of premedical attainment and each of the three steps of the USMLE. The multiple correlation coefficients for these analyses are shown in figure 4.2.

From the results of these analyses we see three patterns:

1. Both the MCAT science scores and the undergraduate science GPA have the
   strongest correlation with the USMLE I score (scientific knowledge), less
   with USMLE II (clinical knowledge), and least with USMLE III (clinical
   skills).
2. For steps I and II of the USMLE, the MCAT science scores have a stronger
   correlation than does the undergraduate science GPA.
3. The MCAT verbal score has the weakest correlation with the USMLE I score,
   more with USMLE II, and most with USMLE III (clinical skills). Among the
   three measures, the MCAT verbal is the strongest predictor of USMLE III.

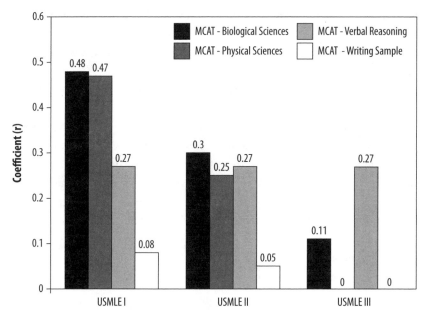

Figure 4.3. Predictive validity coefficients (r) of various measures on USMLE
Step Scores
Source: Data from Donnon et al., 2007

Based on Veloski's research, it appears that it would be optimal to give the MCAT
science scores and the MCAT verbal scores approximately equal weight in the evaluation of applicants to medical school because the combination of the two will give
the strongest prediction of success throughout the various stages of medical education.

Donnon and colleagues reported a similar analysis of the association between
MCAT scores and USMLE scores.[65] They were able to undertake a meta-analysis
of results from 23 separate studies reported between 1991 and 2006, involving more
than 27,000 medical students. Their individual analyses had sample sizes ranging
from 650 for testing the association between individual MCAT test scores with
USMLE Step III scores and 15,000 for testing the association between individual
MCAT test scores with USMLE Step I scores. They did not include undergraduate
GPAs in their analysis. In addition, few of the studies they included in their analysis had data about subject age, gender, or race/ethnicity, so they did not include
these variables. Their results are shown in figure 4.3.

The results of Donnon's study are consistent with those of Veloski's study, with
a few interesting differences. The predictive power of the science MCAT scores is
once again strongest for USMLE I and weakest for USMLE III. The physical sci-

ences MCAT score showed no association with USMLE III. The strongest predictor of USMLE III is once again the MCAT verbal score. In these analyses the MCAT writing sample, added to the MCAT in 1991, had little if any association with performance at any level of medical education.

An earlier report by Hojat and colleagues suggested that, while the writing sample had no association with MCAT science scores or USMLE I scores, better scores on the writing sample were associated with higher scores on the MCAT verbal and on USMLE II.[66] In addition, the authors found that those who did better on the writing sample had higher non-science GPAs as undergraduates but similar science GPAs. The authors were also able to obtain results of a previously validated assessment of clinical skills displayed in the first year of residency, as completed by the residency director. They found that students who did best on the writing sample also scored higher in three areas of clinical skills: data-gathering and processing skills, socioeconomic aspects of patient care, and physician as patient educator. From these analyses the authors reported:

> The findings of the present study confirm the research hypothesis that scores on the Writing Section of the MCAT yield a closer association with measures of clinical competence than with achievement in the basic sciences. . . . Therefore, it can be concluded that the Writing Sample measures a unique skill, different from those measured by the other sections of the MCAT, including the Verbal Reasoning section. It can be speculated that such a unique skill might be attributed more to factors that are not associated with achievement in sciences. Such speculation needs to be verified further by empirical evidence.[67]

Evaluating Medical Students' Performance in an Actual Clinical Setting: The Standardized Patient Examination

In 2004 a new component was added to the USMLE Step II examination: the Standardized Patient Examination (SPE). Similar to the clinical skills assessment reported above by Hojat, this examination was intended to measure the clinical skills of students in their fourth year of medical school by observing them in a series of encounters with patients.[68] In order to standardize the evaluation of students' clinical skills, the NBME hired and trained laypeople to act as patients in order to be able to give a consistent history suggesting a specific medical problem and in some cases to mimic certain physical findings. Over the period of one day, a student evaluates twelve different patients. Each standardized patient is visited by a series of students. Students are scored on a pass/fail basis based on evaluations by the standardized patient and by a trained physician-evaluator. Students must pass this examination in order to be eligible for licensure.

Several individual medical schools have been using standardized patient evaluations for some time as part of the assessment of medical students' clinical skills. In 1992 Vu and colleagues reported on the use of SPEs at the Southern Illinois School of Medicine. Comparing SPE scores with scores on the NBME I and NBME II, they concluded that "the three types of measures did not rank the students similarly and may not have assessed all the same skills."[69] They suggested that faculty use a combination of the three types of examinations to evaluate students. Colliver and colleagues reported that the standardized patient's satisfaction with a student's interpersonal and communication skills during the exam was closely related to the student's skills in history taking and physical examination.[70] Basco and colleagues found little association between the SPE scores of third-year students and those students' undergraduate GPA or MCAT scores.[71] Similarly, Edelstein and colleagues found little or no correlation between SPE scores and either undergraduate GPA or MCAT scores; they did find moderate correlations with USMLE Step I ($r = 0.25$) and Step II ($r = 0.30$).[72]

While the United States adopted the SPE in 2004 as part of the USMLE sequence, the Medical Council of Canada (analogous to the NBME in the U.S.) added an "objective structured clinical examination" (OSCE) to their licensing examination in 1992.[73] The OSCE involves brief encounters with twenty standardized patients and is scored on a numeric basis. In addition to the OSCE, the Canadian licensing examinations include a "Declarative Knowledge" section (MCC Part 1) and a "Clinical Reasoning Skills" section (MCC Part 2). The MCC Parts 1 and 2 are quite similar to the USMLE Steps I and II. Similar to studies in the United States,

- the MCAT Biological Sciences score is correlated with the MCC Part 1 score ($r = 0.19$) but substantially less so with the Part 2 score ($r = 0.03$)
- the MCAT Verbal Reasoning score is correlated both with the MCC Part 1 score ($r = 0.26$) and with the Part 2 score ($r = 0.24$)
- the MCAT Physical Sciences score is correlated neither with the MCC Part 1 score ($r = -0.03$) nor the Part 2 score ($r = 0.02$).[74]

In 2007 Tamblyn and colleagues reported a long-term follow-up of 3,424 physicians in Canada who had taken the OSCE between 1993 and 1996.[75] Comparing the physicians' scores on the OSCE with their MCC scores, they found the correlations shown in table 4.1.

As one might expect, a physician's ability to communicate well with patients is more strongly correlated with the MCC Part 2 than with the MCC Part 1. The data

TABLE 4.1.
Correlation between OSCE scores and scores on Medical Council
of Canada Medical Licensing Examination (MCC) Part 1
(Declarative Knowledge) and Part 2 (Clinical Reasoning Skills)

OSCE Section	MCC Part 1	MCC Part 2
Patient communication	0.10	0.17
Data acquisition	0.21	0.16
Problem-solving	0.36	0.30

Source: Tamblyn et al., 2007.

acquisition and problem-solving sections of the OSCE have the reverse pattern of correlation. The magnitude of the correlation between the communication score and the MCC scores was lower than that of the other parts of the OSCE.

The authors then looked at the frequency of quality of care complaints filed with regulatory authorities against the physicians in the study. They found that "lower [O]CSE communication scores were associated with a higher rate of retained complaints, particularly in the lowest quartile of these scores."[76] In an editorial accompanying the Tamblyn article, Makoul and Curry responded to these results by recommending that, in order to improve quality of care, "initiatives could include more systematically assessing interpersonal skills during the admissions process . . . and ensuring that clinical skills assessments include a communications component."[77]

The SPE and the OSCE appear to offer a valuable additional means of assessing the clinical and professional skills of medical students at the completion of their medical education. As the traditional measures used to evaluate students for admission—science GPA and MCAT scores—appear to have little power to predict the clinical skills measured by the SPE, we will need further research to identify which characteristics of applicants, both cognitive and noncognitive, provide the best prediction of a student's future level of these clinical skills.

A Need to Rethink the Criteria We Use to Select Medical Students

When in the 1920s medical schools first started using measures of premedical performance to sort and select students for admission, the principal concern for admissions officials was to reduce the number of admitted students who failed the medical curriculum. That curriculum had only recently become grounded in science, with nearly all medical schools adopting the four-year, science-based curriculum by 1920. Given the rigor of the science curriculum in the first two years of medical school and the relatively weak premedical preparation in the sciences of many applicants at that time, it is not surprising that as many as one medical student in four failed the first-year curriculum and left medical training. As discussed earlier in this chapter, this loss of students was seen as a costly "wastage," something to be avoided if at all possible. It was for this reason that the Medical Aptitude Test (MAT) was first developed. Used in combination with grades in the premedical sciences, scores on the MAT could predict which students were at the highest risk of failing the first year of medical school.

From the beginning of the period in which the MAT was used, most medical educators fully appreciated that, while a low MAT score predicted the likelihood of failure, it was by no means 100 percent accurate. Experience had shown that substantial numbers of students who were admitted despite low grades or low MAT scores were nonetheless able to complete medical training successfully and become fully qualified physicians. When the MAT was applied increasingly to weed out low-scoring students from the admissions process, educators continued to be aware that a certain percentage of those students denied admission on this basis might have been successful in medical school. The issue was finding the most "efficient" manner in which to apply the achievement-based admissions criteria, with "efficiency" defined as attaining the optimal balance between preventing first-year failure and minimizing the rejection of otherwise qualified applicants.

Following the substantial increase in the number of applicants to medical school that came in the wake of World War II, medical educators were again concerned principally with preventing failure among admitted students. By that time, however, the failure rate of medical students had been reduced substantially. Of all U.S. medical students admitted to medical school between 1949 and 1958, only 9 percent failed to complete medical school. The first-year failure rate during this period averaged between 5 and 7 percent.[78] Despite the markedly reduced failure rate, the use of grades in the premedical sciences and standardized test scores (by then the MCAT was being used) continued to be the principal means by which students were selected for medical school.

Beginning in the 1950s questions arose as to whether likelihood of success in the preclinical sciences taught during the first two years of medical school was either an optimal or an adequate measure. While success in the sciences was certainly important, the likelihood of success as a clinician was at least equally, if not more important. The problem was, though, that the measures used to predict success in the preclinical sciences—premedical science grades and MCAT science scores—had little if any power to predict clinical quality or skills.

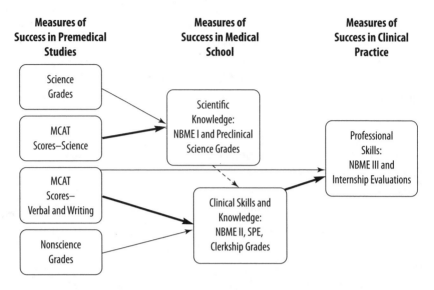

Figure 4.4. Predicting success in medical school and in clinical practice

From a series of research reports, it became apparent that clinical skills reflect a different set of attributes than scientific knowledge and that a different set of factors predict those skills. While premedical science achievement predicts success in the preclinical sciences, it is verbal ability, as measured principally by the MCAT Verbal Reasoning score, that is the strongest predictor of clinical quality. When the SPE was added to the assessment of clinical skills in the USMLE, this conclusion was reinforced. Verbal ability and other humanistic skills are the best predictors of clinical quality, especially the crucially important quality of patient communication. From these research results, it is possible to conceptualize the associations depicted in figure 4.4. The arrows in the figure reflect research about factors shown to be valid predictors, with the width of the arrow representing the strength of the prediction.

Between 2002 and 2007, the number of students graduating from medical schools nationally represented 96.7 percent of the number of students admitted to medical school four years earlier.[79] Of the average of 3.3 percent of entering medical students who failed to graduate, approximately half experienced academic failure during the first two years of school; a substantial share of these students left medical school for personal rather than academic reasons. "Wastage" among first and second year medical students, the principal factor predicted by using premedical science grades and MCAT science scores to rank students for admission, is no longer a serious problem. Nearly every student admitted to medical school will graduate from medical school, barring personal or emotional problems. It no longer seems as appropriate to invest achievement in the premedical sciences with the importance that admissions committees gave them beginning in 1930.

If verbal ability and humanistic skills are the principal predictors of clinical ability and professional skills, as figure 4.4 suggests, it seems only prudent to place more emphasis on measures of these abilities and skills in selecting students for medical school. As studies from the SPE suggest, these abilities and skills reflect both cognitive (i.e., academic achievement) and noncognitive (i.e., personal and psychological characteristics) aspects of medical students. In the following chapter, I examine research on evaluating the noncognitive aspects of premedical and medical students as predictors of professional success.

CHAPTER FIVE

Noncognitive Factors That Predict Professional Performance

Obviously, three requirements are fundamental: mental equipment, physical equipment, and that quality so difficult to define—character.

John Wyckoff, 1927

We are going to be forced to pay more attention to other qualities of character and personality. . . . These things are hard to define and difficult to measure, but they may be the most important factors.

Philip B. Price, 1964

In the previous chapter I traced the origins of the current system of evaluating applicants to medical school based largely on their cognitive abilities, measured as success in the undergraduate premedical sciences. However, beginning more than eighty years ago, medical educators such as those cited above were voicing concerns about including in the evaluation process assessment of noncognitive characteristics such as "character" and "personality." Addressing the Association of American Medical Colleges (AAMC) in 1930, Dr. Edward Thorpe of the University of Pennsylvania Medical School cautioned, "If more courses in chemistry, biology, and physics are needed to prepare students for the medical school curricula of the present and future, what effect has maximum preparation had on students in the past? . . . I have noted with some misgivings the depreciation in that abstract quality called culture in the average applicant for medical training."[1] At that same meeting, E. P. Lyons, dean of the University of Minnesota Medical School, delineated what was meant by the term *culture:* "Culture is the antithesis of specialism, of research, of scholarship. Culture is broad; to the extent that our medical curriculum is narrowing, it is anti-cultural."[2]

Between 1927, when Wyckoff made his comments quoted in the epigraph as part of his research on how to select students for admission to medical school,[3] and 1956, when the AAMC held its training institute titled "The Appraisal of Applicants to Medical School," medical education researchers paid scant attention to including assessment of an applicant's "character" or "culture" as part of the medical school admissions process. As described in the previous chapter, the AAMC's training institute was followed by a shift in the focus of research on predicting the outcomes of medical education. The discussions at the institute were equally as concerned with considering an applicant's intellectual, or cognitive characteristics[4] as they were with considering the non-intellectual, or noncognitive characteristics of applicants.[5] The latter discussion concluded, "It is evident that the so-called nonintellectual characteristics of medical applicants—the elusive personal and social traits and motivational factors—share importance with the more readily measurable intellectual traits in the appraisal of applicants to medical school."[6]

How should one measure in a reliable and valid manner the noncognitive characteristics of an individual interested in a medical career? This question absorbed much of the attention of the conference attendees. The simplest way to address this question was to include a personal interview with the applicant as part of the admissions process—a practice that was becoming increasingly prevalent among medical schools at that time. While the institute participants were in general agreement on the importance of the admissions interview, they nonetheless acknowledged some skepticism about the validity of the interview in evaluating noncognitive attributes: "As long as we have no objective way of determining our criteria for good physicians of whatever variety, and as long as we have no objective ways of evaluating some of the traits that are allegedly prerequisites for becoming a good physician, the interview is the only tool we have for estimating traits."[7] The report of the meeting called for additional research to confirm or support the role of the interview in assessing the noncognitive characteristics of applicants to medical school. This chapter will consider the results of this research.

In addition to using a personal interview to evaluate applicants, two other approaches were discussed at the conference: psychiatric interviews and standardized psychological tests. Dr. Joel Handler reported on the results of psychiatric interviews conducted with more than 500 medical students from three entering classes at the University of Illinois College of Medicine.[8] Dr. Handler and his colleagues had not actually used the results of psychiatric interviews in the admissions process. Rather, they had administered these interviews to incoming students on a voluntary basis (although only two of the more than 500 incoming students declined to be interviewed). Dr. Chandler's findings were not particularly flattering regarding the psychiatric profile of the incoming students: "Our impression was that the majority of the students we saw were quite conformist, emotionally constricted men and women, given to internalizing their hostility either with depressive or compulsive traits for the most part."[9] Chandler's description of the students he interviewed are certainly not what Dr. Wyckoff had in mind when he described "that quality so difficult to define—character."

Regardless of what Dr. Chandler found, it seemed neither practical nor ethical to use a routine psychiatric assessment as a tool with which to evaluate applicants to medical school. However, the use of standardized psychological assessments presented the opportunity to get at many of the characteristics Dr. Chandler was addressing. There was extensive discussion at the AAMC's 1956 meeting of the potential role of psychological tests in improving the admissions process for medical schools. Subsequent to this meeting, the AAMC began its Longitudinal Study, in which researchers administered a battery of psychological tests to entering medical students at 28 different medical schools and then followed these students into their professional careers. Results from this study were in two papers presented to the annual meeting of the AAMC in 1963.

In the first paper, Charles Schumacher of the National Board of Medical Examiners described the purpose of the AAMC's Longitudinal Study as providing an answer to two questions: (1) What are the psychometric tools that will permit medical schools to improve their technique for selecting medical students? and (2) What are the psychometric tools with which medical schools might improve their techniques for counseling and guidance of medical students? Schumacher looked at five different specialty areas in medical practice (general practice, internal medicine, surgery, medical research/teaching, surgical research/teaching), comparing individuals within these groups on three factors: scholastic aptitude, personality characteristics, and biographical histories. He found the specialists engaged in teaching showed higher scholastic aptitude, as measured by their MCAT scores, and personality characteristics consistent with the desire to create new knowledge. By contrast, the practicing physicians, especially the general practitioners, scored lower on the MCAT while showing personality traits that were conducive to "the practical application of knowledge to the everyday problems of patient care, rather than in the creation of new knowledge." To Schumacher it was clear that, upon entering medical school, students displayed personality traits as measured on standardized psychological tests that could be used to predict the type of medical career they would select. Schumacher made no attempt to suggest that one set of personality traits was preferable to another. Rather, he simply confirmed that traits differed in predictable ways among students headed in different career directions.[10]

In the second paper presented at the 1963 meeting, Edwin Hutchins, a researcher from the AAMC, compared the psychological profiles of entering medical students with the profiles of graduating college students in general. He found a series of differences, including the following:

· Medical students scored higher on theoretical and aesthetic scales, suggesting suitability for intellectual pursuits.
· Medical students tended to score higher on scales of individualism and self-sufficiency.
· Medical students scored lower on scales of social and altruistic values.
· Medical students tended to be more conventional, with less need for independence in decision making.[11]

For nearly three decades John Caughey served as associate dean for admissions at Western Reserve University School of Medicine (now Case-Western Reserve). In this capacity he was actively involved in AAMC activities and for a number of years served as chairman of the AAMC's Group on Student Affairs, which had been established as a result of the discussions at the 1956 training institute. In 1966 he reported to the group on the ten-year follow-up of the work on the psychological assessment of medical students and medical school applicants that had been initiated at the 1956 institute. He commented that medical educators continued to do a good job of assuring an adequate level of scientific knowledge of all medical students. However, he was concerned about the relatively little weight admissions committees gave to the "nonintellectual components of medical education, which are of critical importance in the development of the physician."[12] Caughey stressed the importance of personal integrity as a characteristic of at least equal importance as premedical academic attainment in identifying students qualified for the study of medicine. However, medical schools continued to function without a reliable means of assessing integrity. Caughey was also concerned that, on realizing the emphasis medical schools placed on scientific knowledge over noncognitive personal qualities, premedical students would themselves de-emphasize improving those very noncognitive qualities.

In response to the results of the AAMC's Longitudinal Study reported above by Hutchins and with direct reference to Caughey's remarks, Parlow and Rothman reported on an effort at the University of Toronto Faculty of Medicine to incorporate and give added weight in the admissions process to measures of noncognitive characteristics. To do this, they administered a series of psychological tests to incoming medical students over the period 1967–72. They found that by incorporating this dual emphasis in the admissions process they were able to select those students who scored highly on both those cognitive characteristics conducive to academic success and those noncognitive characteristics, such as "nurturance," that are, "the most germane to medical practice."[13]

Haley and Lerner undertook similar research in which they administered a battery of psychological tests to 114 medical students in two successive entering classes at the University of Kentucky College of Medicine. They then followed the students through the first two years of medical school to look for both cognitive (MCAT scores and undergraduate grades) and noncognitive (psychological traits) predictors of academic success. Their findings raise some critical issues: "In general the results indicate that students who do well in the majority of courses . . . tend to have submissive and uncritical attitudes toward authority and a relatively cynical view of human conduct. They are comparatively ambitious to achieve personal, political, or economic power . . . and less socially concerned than students who do less well in these courses."[14] In looking to see which psychological traits were associated with success in the pre-clinical science courses, the authors found that "terms [such] as intelligent, sensitive, or socially concerned . . . either had no association or were negatively associated with the majority of courses."[15]

Turner and colleagues reported on their research at the College of Medicine at Ohio State University in which they administered a series of psychological tests to 50 incoming medical students and then compared the results of these tests with students' performance in a videotaped interaction with a patient.[16] In much the same way that the Standardized Patient Examination would be scored thirty years later, students were rated in three areas of clinical quality: communication skill, interpersonal skill, and physical examination skill. While they found significant positive associations between measured clinical skills and initial psychological measures such as "emotionally stable" and "judgment-perception," they found a significant negative association between clinical skills and MCAT science subtest scores. These results led the authors to encourage the use of psychological tests more broadly in medical schools.

Researchers from the University of California, Berkeley, administered psychological tests on an experimental basis to incoming medical students at the University of California, San Francisco (UCSF), between 1955 and 1967. They then followed these students through medical school to address two questions: (1) Did the results of the psychological tests predict academic performance in medical school? and (2) Did the results of the psychological tests predict failure to graduate? Consistent with previous research on cognitive performance, Gough reported that MCAT science scores and undergraduate science GPA were associated with grades in the first two years of medical school at UCSF, but were "almost completely unrelated to performance in the fourth year and to faculty rating of general and clinical competence." However, those same students who excelled in science as premedical students were found, on the psychological tests, "to be narrower in interests, less adaptable, less articulate, and less comfortable in interpersonal relationships than their lower scoring peers."[17]

In their study of the factors associated with failure to graduate, Gough and Hall found that, of 1,071 incoming medical students at UCSF, 1.6 percent withdrew from school for academic reasons and 3.8 percent withdrew for personal, nonacademic reasons, for an overall failure rate of 5.4 percent. They found that the psychological tests administered at the beginning of school were somewhat better at predicting failure than were the traditional predictors of MCAT scores and premedical grades. Based on this research, they suggested that admissions committees use a combination of cognitive and noncognitive assessments to get a better picture of those students most as risk of failure during medical school.[18]

The results of Gough's research are of particular interest to me because I entered the UCSF medical school as a first-year student in the fall of 1968, the year immediately following Gough's twelve-year study. As a student activist, I was permitted to become the first medical student ever to sit on the UCSF medical school admissions committee, a seat I held from 1968 to 1973. While Gough's work was not published until two years after I left the admissions committee, not once did I hear his results discussed within the committee. The issue of using as part of the admissions process an applicant's noncognitive characteristics as measured on standardized psychological tests was never broached. As far as we were concerned, the principal characteristics qualifying an applicant for admission were high MCAT science scores and high grades in the premedical sciences. The personal interview was useful to flush out more information about an applicant's personality, but it was not used in a standardized way. At least at UCSF at the end of the 1960s, the admissions process paid little attention to the recommendations stemming from the AAMC's 1956 workshop or to Gough's own conclusions that the admissions practices used at that time by UCSF and other medical schools "may be overemphasizing scientific talent and interests and thereby underemphasizing other desirable talents and attributes."[19] A review published in 1989 by Miller and colleagues confirmed that slightly more than half of U.S. medical schools incorporated consideration of noncognitive characteristics into their admissions process but that they did so mostly by following general statements about considering characteristics such as a candidate's honesty, dedication, or consideration for others, without any formal assessment of these traits.[20]

While U.S. medical schools failed to incorporate the standardized assessment of psychological characteristics into their admissions process, at least one school outside the United States did so based on the growing scientific support for such an approach. In 1985 Feletti and colleagues reported on their experience at the Newcastle Medical School in New South Wales, Australia.[21] Students in Australia were accepted into medical school after finishing secondary school in a system of admissions similar to the historic European model. The traditional means of selection was a student's score on a series of standardized academic aptitude examinations. Acknowledging that doubts had been raised over the use of this admissions process, the admissions committee adopted a policy of admitting half of the entering class based on the traditional measures of academic attainment and half of the class based on the results of a series of psychological assessments of students' strengths in areas such as empathy, creativity, response to moral dilemmas, and skills in abstract reasoning (though students admitted based on their psychological characteristics were required also to achieve a certain threshold level of academic attainment). The authors' general conclusion was that the students who were selected based on their psychological profile were equally as successful in medical school as their classmates whose selection was based purely on academic attainment.

Despite the failure of most medical schools to adopt formal psychological assessment as part of the admissions process, a number of researchers in the 1980s and 1990s continued to study the associations between psychological characteristics and medical school performance. For example, in 1987 Aldrich reported a follow-up study of the use of formal psychiatric assessment of incoming medical students, suggesting that such interviews could identify students exhibiting passivity, social isolation, or unusual levels of anxiety or rigidity, and that such students might be at increased risk of failing to graduate for personal rather than academic reasons.[22]

Hojat and colleagues published two papers describing their administration of a series of standardized psychological tests to second-year medical students, then following those students through medical school and into their residency training. Their first analysis compared the use of MCAT scores with the use of the results of the psychological tests to predict grades on the basic sciences examinations in the first two years of medical school, grades on the clinical science examinations in the six core clerkships, and ratings of clinical competence given by the instructor in each of the six core clerkships. The authors found that "the admissions measures and the psychological measures predicted the students' basic sciences and clinical sciences examination grades equally well, but the psychological measures were better predictors of the students' clinical ratings than were the admission measures."[23] When the authors followed the students into their residency, they again found "significant links between selected psychosocial measures and physician clinical competence ratings." After placing their findings in the context of their earlier research and that of others, they suggested, "It is not only mental abilities but also psychological attributes or emotional quotient (EQ) that enhance professional effectiveness above and beyond the well-known concept of intelligence quotient (IQ)."[24]

In 1990 William McGaghie of the University of North Carolina School of Medicine published a two-part review of an extensive literature on the medical school admissions process, paying particular attention to the use of what he called "qualitative variables."[25] Consistent with the other research described in this and previous chapters, McGaghie concluded that there was at best a weak link between a student's academic performance as an undergraduate and his or her achievement across the full medical school experience. Furthermore, he cited considerable evidence that, while medical schools pay what he referred to as "lip service" to the importance of noncognitive attributes such as character, motivation, and personality, they continued to select students for admission based on high MCAT scores and high grades in the premedical sciences: "Despite widespread acknowledgement that qualitative factors are crucial for success as a medical student and physician, the variables are rarely measured or considered when medical schools reach decisions about student admission."[26] McGaghie concluded his analysis by suggesting that, since the time in the 1960s when medical educators first became aware of the value of assessing noncognitive characteristics, there had been little if any progress in actually incorporating formal evaluation of these qualities into the admissions process.

In the last several years, we have continued to see research reports on the importance of noncognitive factors in predicting success in medical school, nearly all consistent with the research that preceded them. Shen and Comrey looked at the medical school experience of 97 economically or socially disadvantaged students who had attended the UCLA school of medicine, confirming that the traditional measures of undergraduate academic performance were associated with academic success in the early years of medical school, while personality characteristics were more predictive of success in the clinical years.[27] Cariaga-Lo and colleagues confirmed that most medical school delays or failures occur in the first two years and that a combination of cognitive and noncognitive measures is best suited to identifying those students who may experience delay or difficulty.[28] Carrothers and colleagues reported testing a new multi-item measure of what they referred to as "emotional intelligence," which, they concluded, "is weakly correlated with indicators of factual knowledge and analytic skills, and strongly correlated with the traditional instrument that measures how well a student will perform the social role of being a physician."[29] Finally, Manuel and colleagues tested whether personality factors were associated with the clinical skills of second year medical students, and were able to confirm such an association.[30]

Success in medical school involves academic success. This has been clear since the 1920s or before. Success in medical school, however, also involves the development and expression of aptitudes that go considerably beyond scholastic aptitude. Only when a student is able to exhibit the full range of requisite aptitudes is she or he fully prepared to become a physician. In 1996 the AAMC initiated a Medical School Objectives Project (MSOP) and charged its participants with identifying those attributes that all medical students should have by the time they have completed training. In 1999 the MSOP Writing Group issued its report, identifying the core attributes students will develop in order to consider their medical education to be a success:

1. *Physicians must be altruistic.* They must be compassionate and empathetic in caring for patients, and must be trustworthy and truthful in all their professional dealings.
2. *Physicians must be knowledgeable.* They must understand the scientific basis of medicine and be able to apply that understanding to the practice of medicine.
3. *Physicians must be skillful.* They must be highly skilled in providing care to individual patients.
4. *Physicians must be dutiful.* They must feel obliged to collaborate with other health professionals and to use systematic approaches for promoting, maintaining, and improving the health of individuals and populations.[31]

The delineation of these requisite attributes provides medical schools with a means of evaluating their own curricula and gauging their own success. While it suggests a framework that might be applied to the selection of students for medical school from the applicant pool, most schools have yet to incorporate formal assessment of the noncognitive characteristics that have been shown to be associated with the full development of these attributes. As early as 1976 a Noncognitive Working Group established by the AAMC had recommended including assessment of a series of noncognitive characteristics in the MCAT. The project was never implemented.[32] In a review of the barriers to incorporating formal assessment of noncognitive characteristics in the admissions process, Albanese and colleagues identified three such barriers: "institutional self-interest, inertia, and philosophical and historical factors."[33]

Medical educators in the United States are not alone in being reluctant to place added emphasis on the assessment of noncognitive characteristics. Reviewing medical education in the United Kingdom, Ferguson and colleagues questioned the traditional emphasis on scholastic attainment and the de-emphasis of noncognitive characteristics: "Previous academic ability, personal statements, references, and interviews are all traditionally used in selection, but how good are they at predicting future performance? Personality and learning style are not traditionally used, but should they be?"[34]

The model of basing admission to medical school on scholastic aptitude, principally in the sciences, evolved in the United States over a period of several decades in an attempt to incorporate the European model of medical education into our own. The growing body of evidence that success in medical education and in medical practice depends on a substantially broader range of factors than scholastic aptitude alone offers us the opportunity to reassess the methods we use to select from among applicants for admission those students best suited to the future practice of medicine. Finding ways to accomplish this goal continues to present substantial challenges, but not necessarily challenges that cannot be overcome.

The Admissions Interview as a Means to Assess the Noncognitive Strengths of Applicants

The AAMC's four-day meeting in 1956 to address "The Appraisal of Applicants to Medical School" looked separately at the appraisal of intellectual characteristics and of "nonintellectual" characteristics. Participants discussed two principal means of evaluating the noncognitive characteristics of medical school applicants: formal psychological tests and admissions interviews. As we have discussed, with rare exceptions psychological tests have not been incorporated into the admissions process in the United States. The admissions interview, however, has been part of that process for several decades. In 1956 all of the 89 medical schools responding to the AAMC's survey about the sources they use for evaluating noncognitive characteristics indicated that they used the personal admissions interview, with 72 percent of the respondents indicating that they relied heavily on the interview in this regard.

Despite the universal use of the admissions interview, the introduction to the report in which these data were presented explicitly acknowledged the dilemma facing the schools: "It is clearly evident that some of the characteristics *valued* most highly by medical schools are those which they have least confidence in evaluating. . . . For the nonintellectual characteristics, there appears to be a negligible correlation between the recognized importance of these factors and the degree of confidence in their evaluation."[35] There was consensus among participants at the meeting that the personal interview had little role in predicting the academic success of medical students in the early years of medical school. Rather, the interview served principally to clarify information in the formal application form and permit the applicant to explain any unusual aspects of the application, to screen for what were referred to as "gross deficiencies in personality and emotional stability," and to gather personal information about the applicant that can be used at the margins of the decision process when there are more applicants who are academically qualified than there are available admissions slots.[36]

Despite acknowledging the importance of predicting success in both the preclinical sciences of medical school and the clinical aspects of medical school, participants were reluctant to use the interview to predict future clinical success for a simple reason: "Before one can test whether the interview can be used to predict future performance of medical applicants, it will be necessary to establish criteria of success in medicine."[37]

Participants in the 1956 meeting held a symposium focused exclusively on "The Interview as One Tool for Selection," with the presentation and discussion of a series of papers. Joseph Zubin, a biometrician, suggested that the purpose of the interview "is to gather information about the candidate's motives, feelings, attitudes, and integrity insofar as they determine his interests in medicine and his ability to deal with peoples."[38] However, Zubin also pointed out some potential problems in using the interview in this manner, principal of which is the "halo effect" by which the interviewer forms a general impression of the interviewee based on information contained in the formal application (e.g., grades, MCAT scores) and allows that general impression to influence his or her assessment of the applicant's noncognitive characteristics as well.

Zubin's paper was followed by one presented by E. Lowell Kelly, a professor of psychology from the University of Michigan. Kelley described his own research and that of others demonstrating that there simply was no evidence of the validity of the interview as a predictor of future performance, either in medical school or in medical practice.[39] Medical schools believed strongly in the utility of the interview, and the longer they used the interview as part of the admissions process the more they tended to believe in them. That belief, however, was not supported by scientific evidence.

Kelley also presented a largely unrelated but nonetheless interesting result from his research on the performance of medical students at the University of Michigan. In evaluating grades throughout the medical school experience, clinical as well as preclinical, he found that "the number of premedical credit hours in inorganic chemistry and in biology submitted by the applicant is negatively correlated with medical school grades."[40] Kelly was one of the first researchers to suggest dual predictive associations for the amount of science a student had included in his or her premedical curriculum: more science predicted better performance in the preclinical sciences of medical school but worse performance in the clinical aspects. We will see this inverse association again in the discussion of the role of empathy in medical school success.

The 1956 meeting called repeatedly for more research on the use of the interview in the medical school admission process. In 1990 Edwards and colleagues published a review of that research. They were able to identify several important trends and results about the role of the interview. While acknowledging the "halo effect" as a potential pitfall, they suggested that the use of structured interviews with training for the interviewers offered a way to avoid that effect. When interviews were appropriately structured, there was "some evidence, albeit imprecise, that the interview actually predicts clinical performance in medical school." To do this best, the interview should de-emphasize information pertaining to academic performance and focus instead on identifying personal characteristics of the applicant such as "leadership, motivation, range of interests, and interpersonal skills." The key to success in this regard is for each medical school to decide for itself what constitutes "success" in medical practice and to look for those noncognitive characteristics that have been shown to be associated with success measured in that way.[41]

In an editorial accompanying the paper by Edwards and colleagues, Thomas Taylor of the University of Iowa College of Medicine expressed skepticism about the role of the interview: "The interview is well entrenched in the admissions process, and it has the validity that comes from habit. Everyone is used to it. It is like an old cat. And like that old cat, it probably will hang around for a while, though nobody can really explain why."[42]

Harasym and colleagues conducted research in which they included some "standardized applicants" in the interview pool at one Canadian medical school. Similar to the standardized patients used as part of medical licensure examinations, the standardized applicants were trained actors enacting scripted roles. Each actor was interviewed by six different interviewers, and the scoring of the interviewers was compared to assess the statistical reliability of the scoring process. The results were not especially encouraging. The researchers found significant variability among the scores of the various interviewers. They did note, however, that the more experienced the interviewer, the more consistent was the scoring.[43]

Despite questions about the reliability of interview scores, Elam and Johnson, in a study of voting patterns in a medical school admissions committee, noted that interview scores had a strong and direct association with the number of supporting votes cast by committee members for an applicant.[44] Also looking at admissions committee voting patterns, Georgesen and colleagues addressed a somewhat different question: for those applicants deemed acceptable but placed on an alternate list pending the results of the first round of offers of admission, what factors are associated with a candidate's position on the alternate list? As admissions officers go down the alternate list as slots open up, an applicant's position on that list can be a key determinant of his or her chances of subsequently being admitted. They found that an applicant's interview scores were the strongest predictor of position on the list, but in a reverse manner. Each applicant had two interview scores. The higher of the two scores had little association with placement on the list, while the lower score had a strong association with placement. Admissions committee members were hesitant to give priority to an applicant with a single low interview score, while paying relatively little attention to a conflicting but higher score.[45]

In sum, it seems that, if done well, an admissions interview can elicit information regarding noncognitive characteristics that is useful in predicting future academic and professional success. To be done well, an interview should be consistently structured so as to elicit the same information across candidates. The interview should be designed to assess those specific noncognitive characteristics thought to be important by the medical school. Interviewers should be trained in its use. When done in this manner, the interview gathers important information that will have a low correlation with traditional measures of cognitive ability, such as premedical sciences grades and MCAT scores, as confirmed by the research of Patrick and colleagues.[46]

The Role of Empathy in Medical Care and in the Selection of Medical Students

Deciding which noncognitive characteristics to assess as part of the admissions process depends on how an admissions committee views the concept of professional success in medicine. The AAMC addressed this issue in a report published in 1984 titled "Physicians for the Twenty-first Century." In the report, a panel of researchers and educators affirmed that "all physicians, regardless of specialty, require a common foundation of knowledge, skills, values, and attitudes." The panel identified one specific attribute as primary: "We believe that every physician should be caring, compassionate, and dedicated to patients."[47] Caring and compassion require empathy—a sense of emotional understanding and connectedness with the patient.

Empathy as an emotional reaction to an interaction or observation has been recognized for more than two centuries as distinct from a cognitive or intellectual reaction to the same situation. Empathy is a concept that can be measured along multiple dimensions, such as concern, adopting another's perspective, and sensing another's distress. Psychologists have been able to develop reliable methods of measuring empathy and have found that it is a characteristic largely independent of scholastic attainment. When researchers in one study administered psychological tests to college students in an introductory psychology course, they found that the various measures of empathy had little if any correlation with measures of cognitive ability such as the subscales of the Scholastic Aptitude Test.[48]

In 1978 David Kupfer, a faculty psychiatrist, and Frances Drew, the student affairs dean, both at the University of Pittsburgh School of Medicine, published a provocative article regarding the personality characteristics of medical students. The authors acknowledged the growing body of research at the time suggesting that MCAT scores and grades in the premedical sciences, while having substantial power to predict academic performance early in medical school, had little power to predict performance in the clinical years. In their own school they had administered a standardized instrument measuring empathy to more than 500 students and then looked for correlations between MCAT scores and empathy scores. They found few significant relationships, with those that did reach statistical significance being fairly small in magnitude. They concluded that empathy and other similar personality characteristics reflect dimensions that are separate and distinct from cognitive ability. Given the importance of empathy and the large number of applicants who have the academic strength to succeed in medical school, they suggested that medical schools look first for those applicants who are high on both dimensions: cognitive ability and empathy.[49]

Branch and colleagues describe medical students' own perspectives on empathy, using students' written narratives of their interactions with patients. In many of these narratives, students acknowledged the critical importance of connecting with their patients empathetically: "To a remarkable degree, the medical students put themselves in their patients' shoes . . . the students' learning to understand patients' experiences through empathy often improved their relationships with patients."[50] There is another thing to be learned from reading these narratives. Not only do students recognize the value of their own ability to empathize with patients, they also readily recognize a lack of empathy or compassion on the part of their student colleagues or the practicing physicians with whom they work and the adverse effects of such a lack.

Empathy is "the ability to understand another person's emotional or life experience; it is to share those emotions' content but not their intensity." Using this definition, E. R. Marcus links empathy with the distinct but related quality of humanism and identifies them as capacities that are critical to the practice of medicine. From Marcus's perspective, empathy reflects an ability, and humanism an attitude. Unfortunately, based on Marcus's experience training medical students and residents in psychiatry, the experience of medical school often is inimical to the development of empathetic ability and a humanistic attitude: "Constant picayune testing, a threatening academic atmosphere, and a competitive curve grading system increase student competition and student anxiety, and reinforce the grandiose 'must master it all' defense. The bigger this defense, the bigger the inevitable crash and the greater the resultant humiliation and anger. The result is a tough emotional crust and marked disidentification with patients: in distancing themselves from their own victimization by the curriculum, students distance themselves from the victims of illness." Marcus suggests that what he refers to as "the rites of passage" of medical school delay the final emotional maturation of the physician until after he or she has completed residency training. This maturation process takes place unconnected to any formal educational process and is subject to variation among individuals.[51]

Whatever the level of empathy with which students enter medical school, research suggests that level will decline over the course of medical education. Diseker and Michielutte assessed students' empathy during the first week of medical school and at the end of the fourth year. Using an empathy scale derived from the California Personality Inventory (CPI), a well-established and previously validated personality assessment, they found a decline in the average level of empathy over the four-year period. In their study, empathy correlated negatively with MCAT scores.[52]

West and colleagues, using a different measurement instrument, evaluated the level of empathy and the level of medical knowledge of entering residents in an internal medicine residency program. They then repeated these assessments at the beginning of the second year. Over the period of one year, these residents demonstrated an increase in their level of medical knowledge but a decrease in their level of empathy. In discussing the implications of their results for the broader process of medical education, the authors concluded "that the core competencies [medical knowledge and empathy] represent separate domains of skill/expertise that develop independently . . . our findings confirm the importance of measuring each domain of competency separately."[53]

Might the rites of passage inherent to medical education, identified above by Marcus, actually begin well before medical school, in the early parts of premedical education? "Constant picayune testing, a threatening academic atmosphere, and a competitive curve grading system," the factors described above by Marcus as impeding the development of empathy, also characterize the early premedical experience, as our interviews with premedical students at Stanford and UC Berkeley, described in the first chapter, so clearly indicate. The academic and personal strengths necessary to succeed in a highly competitive premedical curriculum might be contrary to those strengths that support the development of empathetic ability. Could it be that success in the premedical and preclinical sciences is negatively associated with empathy? This question was addressed by Peter Tutton, a member of the medical faculty at Monash University in Australia.[54]

The medical school at Monash University has a six-year curriculum similar to the historic European model of medical education, with students entering after high school. During the first three years, incoming students study the premedical sciences, with completion of the preclinical sciences and clinical training in the final three years. Tutton administered the CPI to 133 incoming students. He then followed the students through their first three years, comparing their grades in the sciences to their scores on the various scales of the CPI. He found a consistent pattern of correlations.

The principal type of examinations used in the sciences at Monash University involves multiple choice questions (MCQs). Success in MCQs in the sciences was significantly correlated with three of the various personality scales measured by the CPI: empathy, dominance, and internality. The correlation with empathy was a negative one, with a correlation coefficient of −0.36. The better students did on the their science exams through their first three years of college, the lower was their empathy score on entering college. Conversely, those students with the highest empathy as measured by the CPI tended to do worst in their science examinations. The correlation with the scale of dominance was also negative (−0.32), while that with the scale of internality was positive (+0.30).

As explained by the author, a high score on the internality scale, as students who were successful in their MCQs tended to get, suggests that a student may be "shy," "submissive," "withdrawn," or "awkward and ill at ease socially," characteristics the author suggests are "the antithesis of what most of us would want in a clinician." Summarizing his results, Tutton further suggests that "students with high achievement in many components of the curriculum tend to have personality profiles that seem inappropriate for their chosen careers as physicians."[55]

For more than a century, success in the premedical sciences of chemistry, biology, and physics has been seen as a necessary precursor to success in medical school and ultimate success as a physician. Since the 1920s success in the premedical sciences, as measured by undergraduate grades and MCAT scores, has been the principal means of sorting medical school applicants to identify those who are "fit to study medicine," as described Daniel Coit Gilman in 1878. The results of the work by Marcus and Tutton seem to suggest that selecting students based on their success in the premedical sciences may select against students who excel in empathy and humanism, characteristics that are equally important as, if not more important than, cognitive ability in the sciences.

One's overall level of ability does not manifest itself in a single way and cannot be measured along a single axis. Lubinski suggests that there are at least three dimensions to ability: quantitative ability, spatial ability, and verbal ability.[56] Within individuals, different combinations of these three dimensions will be manifested as different proficiencies and proclivities. An individual who excels in one dimension of ability is not more intelligent than someone who excels in another. The concept of general intelligence is reflected in the combination of the three dimensions. Lubinski describes how these various abilities may affect educational outcomes: "People do not select educational tracks and occupations randomly. They do so, at least in part, on the basis of stable features of their personality, which include their specific abilities."[57]

A highly intelligent individual who scores higher in quantitative ability may likely be more comfortable in areas such as math and science; one who scores higher in verbal ability may instead be drawn to social science or the humanities. Conversely, a more verbally oriented person who, for whatever reason, begins his or her education in a scientific field may be more likely to shift out of that field to one that is more compatible with his or her inherent intellectual strengths. A series of research studies, using a unique tool to measure individual differences, confirmed this tendency to shift one's area of study in the face of a mismatch of cognitive style.

Over a period of more than thirty years, Herman Witkin, a psychological researcher working with the Educational Testing Service, studied a phenomenon he referred to as "field dependence" and its association with educational preferences and success. To measure field dependence, a subject sits before a computer screen in a darkened room. On the screen is a quadrilateral figure that looks like a rectangle placed vertically in space but is actually tilted very slightly off vertical. Within the figure is a line that is clearly tilted off vertical. Using a control stick that rotates the line on its center, the subject is asked to reposition the line so as to place it in the vertical position. The question under study is, does the subject ignore the figure and place the line truly vertical, or does the subject use the figure as a field of reference, positioning the line parallel to the figure rather than truly vertical? By repeating the test with a more highly skewed figure, the researchers determine how far off vertical they can position the quadrilateral before the subject ignores it and positions the line independently in space. Those who follow the figure in positioning the line are "field-dependent," while those who tend to ignore the figure are "field-independent."

In their research, Witkin and colleagues followed more than 1,500 entering college students, administering the test and assessing their field dependence/independence at the time they entered college. They then followed these students through the four years of college and into either their work or their graduate education. They arrived at three principal conclusions:

1. Field-independent students tended to select an undergraduate major in the natural sciences or math.

2. Field-dependent students tended to major in education or related social sciences.

3. Either field-dependent students who initially selected a science/math major or field-independent students who initially selected an education/social science major were significantly more likely to change majors than students whose initial selection of a major matched their field dependency score.[58]

There has been debate among psychologists as to whether field dependence actually reflects a form of cognitive ability rather than simple visual tendencies unrelated to measures of intelligence.[59] However, some of Witkin's research results apply specifically to premedical students. Among Witkins research subjects were a substantial number of students who declared an interest in premedical studies early in their college career. (Since Witkin conducted his research at a time when fewer than 10 percent of medical students were female, he only reported results for males.) Consistent with conclusion (3) above, premedical students who were field-independent were significantly more likely to remain in premedical studies and subsequently to apply to medical school than were field-dependent students.

From other research he had done, Witkin was able to compare the personality characteristics of people who were field-dependent or -independent. The difference in personality profiles holds particular relevance to our discussion of the strengths and abilities we look for in physicians. As summarized by Witkin,

> Field-dependent people are more attentive to social cues than are field-independent people. Field-dependent people have an interpersonal orientation: They show strong interest in others, prefer to be physically close to people, are emotionally open, and gravitate towards social situations. Field independent people have an impersonal orientation: They are not very interested in others, show both physical and psychological distancing from people, and prefer nonsocial situations. Finally, field-dependent and field-independent people are different in an array of characteristics that make it likely that field-dependent people will get along better with others.[60]

While acknowledging the debate over Witkin's work, it is hard not to see its relevance to premedical education and to the process by which we select those students best suited to become physicians. Tutton's comments cited above, "that students with high achievement in many components of the [premedical] curriculum tend to have personality profiles that seem inappropriate for their chosen careers as physicians,"[61] appear also to apply to the process by which field-independent students tend to stay in premedical education and enter medicine, while their field-dependent classmates tend to drop out of premedical education and enter other fields.

Whether it is the ability to be emotionally open and comfortable in social situations or the ability to empathize and show compassion, it should be clear that those with a higher level of ability in these areas will be perceived in a better light by their patients than those with less ability. Similarly, when they are evaluated by medical school faculty regarding their clinical skills, those who score higher on scales of empathy will also score higher on assessments of interpersonal skills when working with patients in a clinical context. This association was confirmed by two recent research studies. Hojat and colleagues from Jefferson Medical College administered what they referred to as the Jefferson Scale of Physician Empathy to 371 third-year medical students and then compared the students' empathy scores with a global rating of their clinical competence provided by the faculty in their third-year clinical clerkships. The authors found a significant positive association between the two scores.[62] Similarly, Stratton and colleagues administered a psychological assessment to 165 third-year medical students at the University of Kentucky and then compared these results with the students' performance on a required comprehensive clinical performance examination involving a series of twelve encounters with standardized patients. As described by the authors, "Significant associations were found between the standardized patients' rating of students' communication abilities and their scores on one [emotional intelligence] and two empathy subscales."[63]

Consistent with our discussions above, professionalism for a physician implies both a certain level of cognitive ability in the sciences and a parallel, but distinct, ability in establishing a humanistic connection with patients. This brings up an obvious question: If medical students, selected principally on their proven cognitive abilities in the sciences, tend to be weaker in empathy, can they be taught how to feel and display empathy? This question has been addressed by a number of researchers.

Poole and Sanson-Fisher studied the effects of explicit empathy training on medical students in Australia. As described above, Australian students undergo a six-year medical curriculum, with the final three years completing the preclinical sciences and providing clinical education. The researchers administered formal empathy training to a group of 25 students selected randomly from a group of 45 entering the final three-year curriculum. They were able to identify clear improvement in empathetic ability immediately following the training: "Prior to training they had been hesitant, frequently avoiding emotional topics and tending to dominate the interaction; this changed following training . . . students permitted patients to do most of the talking and encouraged emotional expression; their responses generally indicated understanding and concern for patients." However, by the end of their clinical training, that empathetic behavior in the study subjects had decreased significantly and was only marginally better than the control group, leading the authors to conclude that "the educational experience during the clinical years appears to negate to some extent the earlier training."[64]

One has to question whether the students in the study by Poole and Sanson-Fisher were actually being taught to feel empathy, rather than being taught to act in an empathetic manner without actually personally experiencing empathy. Rees and Knight suggest that, in evaluating professionalism among physicians, we distinguish between attitudes and behaviors. One who acts compassionately does not necessarily feel compassion.[65]

Whether patients can distinguish between compassionate or empathetic behavior that does not have an actual underpinning in true compassion or empathy and behavior that stems from innate empathy remains an open question. Benbassat and Baumal suggest that there is value in teaching students to act empathetically, even if they do not experience true empathy: "We believe that the ability to encourage a patient to convey his distress is a teachable skill, while the subsequent steps are mainly related to the personality traits of each individual student." They emphasize the importance of teaching patient-centered interviewing skills and strengthening the student-physician/patient relationship by restructuring clinical teaching to permit the development of longer-term relationships between the student and the patient. However, the authors discourage the assessment of empathy as part of the admissions process because, "Even if admissions committees could identify an ability to empathize among entry-level medical students, the hospital environment would most likely eradicate this ability."[66]

In their analyses, these authors acknowledge the previous research demonstrating that medical students' level of empathy as measured on standardized psychological instruments declines throughout the process of medical education. A recent paper by Newton and colleagues confirms this finding. They distinguish between "vicarious empathy," in which a student has a genuinely visceral response to a patient or a situation, and "role-playing empathy," in which a student is taught to act in an empathetic manner without experiencing the true sensation. Using the Balanced Emotional Empathy Scale instrument, they tracked 419 entering medical students at the University of Arkansas for Medical Sciences, spread across four entering classes. They administered the Empathy Scale at the beginning of each of the four years of medical school and found consistent declines over time. The decline was particularly steep following the first year and the third year of school. Interestingly, while all students showed nearly parallel declines in empathy over time, those students choosing to go into the more patient-oriented fields of internal medicine, family medicine, obstetrics-gynecology, pediatrics, and psychiatry both entered school with higher levels of empathy and maintained higher levels over time than their classmates who chose more technically oriented specialties.[67]

Howard Spiro of the Yale University School of Medicine published an insightful commentary in 1992 about the role of empathy in medical education and medical practice. His comments were not particularly complementary toward the dominant model of medical education: "As I know them, college students start out with much empathy and genuine love—a real desire to help other people. In medical school, however, they learn to mask their feelings, or worse, to deny them. They learn detachment and equanimity. The increased emphasis on molecular biology to the exclusion of the humanities encourages students to focus not on patients, but on diseases."[68]

Writing in 1983, Gregory Pence, a professor of philosophy and medical ethicist and a faculty member at the University of Alabama Birmingham School of Medicine, emphasized the importance of compassion in medical practice. Referring to the work of Aristotle, he stressed the importance for the physician of developing a sense of intimacy with a patient, intimacy that is "built on related moral qualities between listener and sufferer of trust, honesty, and the time and willingness to listen." Pence shares the skepticism voiced above by Spiro:

> The view [among medical educators] seems to be that the primary goal of medical training is to produce scientifically competent physicians and, as for compassion, well, it will be picked up by "osmosis" (perhaps "perfusion" would be more exact). . . .
>
> Compassion in undergraduates is notoriously difficult to discover or measure, especially in the brief, episodic encounters of mass education between professor and student where future requests for recommendations may lurk in a student's mind. *But even if* compassion could be accurately identified in undergraduates, the crucial problem remains of the great power of medical education to eradicate compassion.[69]

Coulehan and Williams argue that certain students enter medical school with a "natural immunity" to the tacit, implicit forces within medical education that lead to a loss of empathy among medical students over time. Despite the dehumanizing atmosphere of medical school, these "immunized" students "progress through medical school and postgraduate training while maintaining, even nourishing, an altruistic professional persona." The authors suggest that, if it were possible to measure this natural immunity as part of the admissions process, we could avoid the current skewing that favors "individuals who might turn into good scientists or technicians, but who have two strikes against them when it comes to becoming compassionate physicians."[70]

Psychologists will continue to debate whether qualities such as compassion and empathy are innate or can be learned. They will continue to differentiate between acting in an empathetic manner and genuinely feeling the quality of empathy. We can be sure, though, that psychologists, and for that matter philosophers as well, will generally agree that empathy forms a crucial underpinning for competence and professionalism on the part of physicians. The ability to feel empathy is not measured by the MCAT and is not reflected by grades in the premedical sciences—that is, unless the research of Tutton and Witkin, described above, is accurate and the ability to succeed in the premedical sciences is *inversely* related to one's natural empathic abilities and sensitivities. If it were the case that, by selecting students for medical school based on the paradigm of premedical education established more than a hundred years ago, we are selecting *against* those students who are strongest in empathy and *for* those students who are weakest, we would be making a fundamental error. Quoting again from Kupfer's research from 1978, "One interpretation of these findings would be that those ideal attributes found in the 'good physician' are derived from more than one dimension. . . . Therefore, identification of students who have both high MCAT scores and high empathy scores might represent one approach in predicting which students will make the best clinicians."[71]

The Need to Develop a Multidimensional Model of Medical School Admissions

We began this chapter with two quotations made nearly forty years apart yet concurring on the importance of both cognitive and noncognitive qualities in medical education and medical practice. By tracing more than forty years of research that followed the more recent of the quotations, we have found substantial support for this concept. Whether it is the "good physician" referred to by Kupfer or the ideal clinician described by Tutton, he or she will have at least two characteristics: an adequate knowledge of the scientific principles on which medical practice is based and the personal qualities such as character, empathy, and compassion that are requisite for optimal competence as a clinician.

In the MCAT we have a reliable and well-validated means of measuring the scientific knowledge gained from premedical education. As described in the previous chapter, performance on the biological sciences and to a lesser extent on the physical sciences component of the MCAT is a reasonably accurate predictor of future

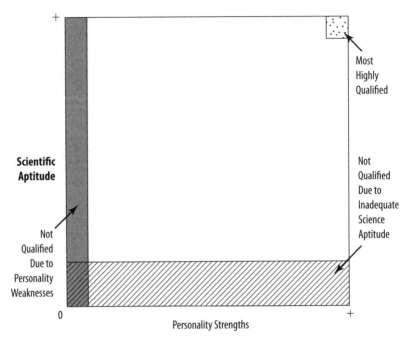

Figure 5.1. A two-dimensional approach to evaluating qualifications for admission to medical school

performance in the preclinical sciences of medical school. These measures of science aptitude, however, tell us little about a student's future performance as a clinician.

The admission interview, if done well, gives us some guidance about an applicant's noncognitive strengths and weaknesses but is unable to provide an accurate prediction of a student's future ability to communicate with patients and to gain their trust through the intimacy afforded by empathy and compassion. Clearly, we need ongoing research on how best to measure these noncognitive aspects of an applicant's qualifications to be selected to enter medical school. However, for the purpose of discussion, let us assume that we have developed a measure of an applicant's personality that is equally reliable and equally valid as the MCAT is in assessing scientific aptitude. How would we use these two measures of an applicant's qualifications? The research cited above suggests that they need to be approached as dimensions that are largely independent. Using these two measures, we could therefore place applicants somewhere in a two-dimensional grid of qualification such as that depicted in figure 5.1.

In figure 5.1, the vertical axis represents a continuous scale of scientific aptitude, evaluated by measures such as the MCAT score or premedical science grades. The horizontal axis represents a continuous scale of personality strengths, assuming we could eventually develop such a measure. The area within the square represents the pool of applicants to medical school. Within this pool there will be some people who simply are not qualified, due to gross inadequacies in their science preparation. These are represented by the diagonally shaded box long the horizontal axis. No matter how great the strength of their personality, these applicants are likely to be unprepared to undertake the study of medicine. While some of these students might eventually succeed in the first two years of medical school, the probability is high that many of them would fail one or more of their preclinical science courses. It was this population that the MCAT was first developed to identify, as described in the previous chapter.

Similarly, there is a somewhat narrower shaded box along the vertical axis, representing those applicants with shortcomings in one or more aspects of their personality that disqualify them for medical practice. While some of these students could possibly complete medical school and become medical researchers with little patient contact, their personality weaknesses make them inappropriate for working with patients. Through the admissions interview and information provided by premedical advisors, these students also need to be identified.

In the upper right corner of figure 5.1 is a smaller, lightly shaded box, representing those medical school applicants who score the highest on both scientific aptitude and strength of personality. Clearly these are the applicants medical schools want the most. They have the firmest grounding in science, and we can reliably predict that they will be seen by their patients as representing the highest level of medical professionalism. Of course, the number of applicants represented by this small box is inadequate to fill the entering class of all the medical schools in the country. How should we expand the box of qualified applicants to a size sufficient to fill the entering class? There are two ways to do this: the way we have been doing it for nearly a hundred years, represented by figure 5.2, and an alternative model, represented by figure 5.3 and based on the realization that we need to evaluate the fitness of an applicant to study medicine using at least two equally important dimensions of quality.

Since the 1920s, when for the first time the number of applicants to medical schools exceeded the number of available places in the first-year class, we have used scientific aptitude as a nearly continuous measure of an applicant's fitness to study medicine. Premedical performance in chemistry, biology, and physics is the principal measure admissions committees have used to rank-order applicants. Extracurricular activities, comments of the premedical advisor, and results of the admission interview provided additional information at the margins. Despite a widespread

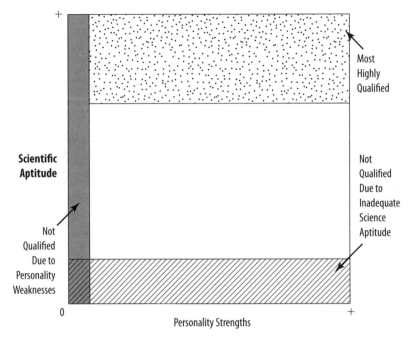

Figure 5.2. The traditional approach to evaluating qualifications for admission to medical school

recognition that character traits such as empathy and compassion play a major role in medical professionalism and the quality of care, the absence of a reliable means of assessing these characteristics left admissions committees little choice but to select those students who were the least likely to fail the preclinical sciences classes encountered in the first two years of medical school—the traditional measure of fitness to study medicine.

The research described in this chapter, however, suggests a fundamental weakness in this approach. Fitness to study medicine is determined by a combination of an applicant's scientific aptitude and his or her personality strengths. Only by including both dimensions in the evaluation process can we get the most complete picture of an applicant's qualifications.

Figure 5.3 provides an alternative approach to expanding our concept of "fit to study medicine." Beginning in the upper-right corner of the diagram, it identifies the set of most highly qualified applicants, but not as a horizontal rectangle using scientific aptitude as means of ranking applicants. Instead, it expands the area of the pool by maintaining the shape of an isosceles triangle, moving down each axis equally and thereby giving equal weight to an applicant's scientific aptitude and his

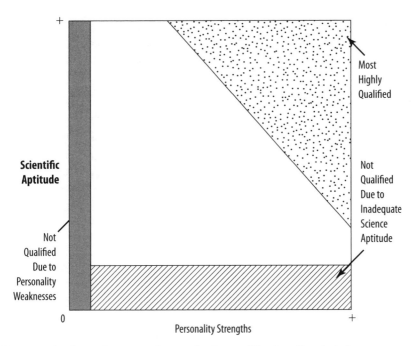

Figure 5.3. An alternative approach to evaluating qualifications for admission to medical school

or her personality strengths. Under this alternative model, there are some applicants who would be admitted to medical school who would not have been admitted under the traditional model—those with relatively lower scientific aptitude but relatively greater personality strength. Conversely, there are some applicants who would have been admitted under the traditional model but who would be denied admission under this model—those applicants who are relatively higher in scientific aptitude but with relatively weaker personality strength.

Which model would produce better physicians? Could we trust as our physician someone who got a B in organic chemistry in college, when we might instead have a physician who got an A? Would a 10 on the biological sciences portion of the MCAT mean that a physician is not as qualified as his or her colleague who got a 12?

Research suggests that patients will tend to put aside these questions and ask instead, "Can I trust my physician? Can she or he *really* understand what it feels like to be sick or injured?" For most patients, that is what makes a good physician.

No matter how much we agree that personality and strength of character are important in selecting students for medical school, we still don't have a means of assessing these noncognitive qualities in a way that is both reliable and feasible. However, we can address the common concern that de-emphasizing academic performance in the premedical sciences will weaken the clinical and professional capabilities of the physicians we train. By looking at research reporting the outcomes of programs that have placed less emphasis in the admission process on attainment in the premedical sciences, we can determine what effect such nontraditional approaches have had. These programs are of two general types: those specifically intended to increase the ethnic diversity of the medical profession, and those that have adopted a nontraditional approach to medical education without ethnic diversity as a singular goal. I discuss these programs in the following chapters.

CHAPTER SIX

Efforts to Increase the Diversity of the Medical Profession

The 1950 graduating class of U.S. medical schools included 55 black students, 8 Latino students, and 1 Native American student, representing about 1 percent of graduates nationally.[1] By 1968, the number of graduates from these underrepresented minority groups had risen to 3.6 percent of all medical students. However, more than half of these URM graduates were enrolled at either Howard University College of Medicine or Meharry Medical College, schools founded to educate black physicians.[2] Among other U.S. medical graduates, fewer than 2 percent were from URM groups.

By 1980, largely the result of affirmative action programs initiated in the late 1960s and early 1970s, students from URM groups had grown to 8.4 percent of medical graduates nationally and included 704 black students, 473 Latino students, and 40 Native American students.[3] By relaxing to a certain extent the stringent premedical requirements that had existed for decades, U.S. medical schools were able to evaluate affirmative action applicants using a somewhat different metric than that used for other applicants, thereby substantially increasing the racial and ethnic diversity of medical graduates and ultimately of the U.S. medical profession.

In 1966 the University of California (UC) opened a new medical school at its Davis campus. Consistent with the affirmative action policies nationally and with policies at other UC campuses, the UC Davis medical school set aside 15–20 percent of its admission slots for URM students and created a special admissions committee to fill these. Using traditional measures of academic performance coupled with an assessment of applicants' noncognitive strengths, the medical school was able to accept the best of the URM applicants for the URM-designated slots and the best of the non-URM applicants for the remainder.

Allan Bakke was a white male in his early thirties who applied to the UC Davis medical school in 1973. As a white student, his application was reviewed by the main admissions committee. Based both on his age (relatively older than his fellow non-URM applicants) and his grades and MCAT scores (relatively lower than his fellow non-URM applicants), he did not receive an offer of admission. Bakke applied again in 1974 and again was rejected. In that same application cycle, the special admissions committee admitted URM candidates who had somewhat lower MCAT scores and premedical grades than Bakke's. Bakke sued UC Davis for racial discrimination. His case was eventually heard by the U.S. Supreme Court, which in 1978 found for Bakke.[4] The court determined that the medical school's allocation of a fixed number of slots for URM students created a type of racial quota that is prohibited by the Constitution. Bakke was admitted to the UC Davis medical school and, despite his relatively low grades and MCAT scores, successfully completed his training.

The effect of the Bakke case on the subsequent medical school admission of URM students is clear. After increasing sharply between 1970 and 1982 (students graduating in 1982 were admitted to medical school in 1978, the year of the Bakke decision), the number of URM graduates of U.S. medical schools remained essentially flat for the next decade.[5]

In the decade leading up to the Bakke case, hundreds of URM applicants were admitted to medical school despite somewhat weaker premedical preparation in the sciences as measured by grades and MCAT scores. Did these students with lower grades and MCAT scores turn out to be weaker medical students? What was the impact of affirmative action policies on professional quality—did affirmative action students turn out to be less competent as physicians? These questions were raised repeatedly in the decade of race-based affirmative action and in the decades following the Bakke decision.

Evans and colleagues addressed these questions in their analysis of the effect of the affirmative action program at Case Western Reserve School of Medicine (CWR). Before 1970, CWR had admitted few URM students, typically fewer than 2 percent of any entering class. Beginning in 1970, CWR began to admit substantially more URM students, many of whom had lower grades and MCAT scores than the non-URM students who were admitted. Evans and colleagues evaluated the performance of 43 of the 66 URM students admitted between 1970 and 1973 on a comprehensive examination given to all medical students at the end of the first year.[6] Consistent with the research described in chapter 4, affirmative action students, many of whom had lower MCAT scores, tended also to score lower on the first-year medical school exam. The researchers also looked at the scores of 26 of these students on the NBME-I licensure examination given at the end of the second year of medical school. Again consistent with earlier research, the URM students with lower MCAT scores tended to score lower on the NBME exam.

However, the authors found no association between the affirmative action students' undergraduate grades and either of these exam scores. Rather than grades, the selectivity of the college or university from which the student graduated, measured on a numeric scale called the Astin index, was found to have a significant association with success on these exams, leading the authors to comment that "the single most valuable criterion for prediction of success among minority medical students at CWR is the competitiveness of the undergraduate college attended as measured by the Astin index."[7] Those URM students coming to CWR from less-competitive colleges were at "significant risk for having academic problems," although the authors emphasized that many of the URM students from these less-competitive colleges were nonetheless able to successfully complete the first two years of medical school and move into their clinical training, where they had much less difficulty.

Addressing these same questions in the decade following the Bakke decision, Dawson and colleagues looked at performance on the NBME-I exam for more than 30,000 students who took the exam in 1986, 1987, or 1988.[8] About 9 percent of these students were from URM groups. In their analysis, the authors were able to include each student's MCAT scores, undergraduate grades, gender, and racial/ethnic group. They found two consistent patterns of association: URM students had lower NBME-I scores than non-URM students; and women had lower scores than men, regardless of race/ethnicity. When the authors then controlled for MCAT scores and undergraduate grades, they found that the difference in NBME-I scores between URM and non-URM students was greatly reduced; however, the difference between men and women remained. For some reason women of any race or ethnicity tended to score lower on the exam regardless of MCAT scores and undergraduate grades, while URM students' scores were largely predicted by these measures.

Based on the results of these studies, one can reasonably conclude that URM students with lower MCAT scores and undergraduate grades admitted to medical school as part of affirmative action programs would, on average, score lower in the first two years of medical school. However, Dawson was careful to point out that attaining lower scores in the first two years of medical school did not necessarily imply lower clinical quality for these URM students once medical education was completed. She cautioned, "Few studies of physician performance in practice settings have been reported, and comparisons of examination results with performance in medical school, residency training, and practice are clearly needed. . . . [T]ests of knowledge base cannot assess many important clinical skills."[9]

How did URM students, admitted under affirmative action programs despite relatively low grades and MCAT scores, ultimately perform in clinical practice settings? The answer to this question is crucial to defining the ultimate effect that affirmative action programs had on clinical and professional quality. A series of studies has given us a fairly clear answer.

Keith and colleagues analyzed data on all U.S. medical graduates in 1975, looking at how URM students, most of whom were admitted to medical school as part of affirmative action programs, compared to non-URM students in choice of specialty, board certification rates, practice location, and patient populations served.[10] They identified several key findings:

- More URM students (12%) than non-URM students (6%) practiced in locations designated as "health manpower shortage areas" by the federal government.
- More URM students (55%) than non-URM students (41%) chose primary care specialties.
- URM physicians were more likely to treat poor patients, minority group patients, and patients on Medicaid.
- Fewer URM students (48%) than non-URM students (80%) were board certified in their specialty ten years following graduation.

The authors questioned whether the lower rate of board certification among URM physicians might be related to the finding that these physicians tended to treat more poor patients and patients on Medicaid, since board certification "is relatively unimportant in the medical marketplace in which they practice."[11]

Davidson and Montoya also addressed this issue in a study of URM and non-URM students graduating from medical schools in California in either 1974 or 1975. They confirmed that, as with the national sample in the study by Keith and colleagues, the URM graduates in California were more likely to practice in a health manpower shortage area and more likely to provide care to patients who were poor, minority, or on Medicaid.[12] In a follow-up study, the authors found that, 12–13 years after graduation, fewer URM students (64%) than non-URM students (90%) were board certified in their specialty. To determine the reason for the lower rate of board certification among URM graduates, they conducted a phone survey of the physicians who were not board certified, both URM and non-URM, and asked them the reason for their lack of board certification. The authors found no difference in the responses given by the URM physicians and the non-URM physicians, reporting that "their responses generally indicated that they perceived no benefit to their practice to compensate for the extra effort needed to attain board certification."[13]

Indeed, for the first eight years of my career as a physician (1974–1982), I saw no need to become board certified. I practiced as a solo primary care physician in a rural, health manpower shortage area. Since I was the only physician within a 20-mile radius, most of my patients were not concerned that I was not board certified.

It was only when I moved my practice to a large managed care organization in an urban setting that I perceived the need to become board certified and took the steps necessary to obtain that certification.

Perhaps the most convincing study of the effect of affirmative action programs on clinical and professional quality was reported by Davidson and Lewis.[14] They were able to identify all students admitted to the UC Davis School of Medicine between 1968 and 1987 who did not meet the ordinarily applied minimum academic standards required for admission. Such students admitted between 1968 and 1978 (the year of the Bakke decision) would have been admitted mostly under the school's affirmative action program. Students admitted between 1978 and 1987 had been considered on a case-by-case basis and offered admission if special circumstances warranted an offer of admission despite substandard grades or MCAT scores. The 356 students admitted in this manner made up 20 percent of the 1,784 students admitted to the medical school during the period of 1968–87.

For each of the special-admit students, the researchers were able to randomly identify a matched regular-admit student for comparison. They then compared the special-admit students with the regular-admit students in a number of areas. The differences identified below were statistically significant, unless otherwise noted.

- *URM status.* 152 of the 356 special-admit students (42.7%) were from URM groups; 58 of all regular-admit students for the period (4%) were from URM groups.
- *Undergraduate grades.* The special-admit students had an average undergraduate GPA of 3.06 on a 4-point scale; the regular-admit students had an average GPA of 3.50.
- *MCAT scores.* The special-admit students entering between 1968 and 1981 had a mean MCAT score (old MCAT) of 544; the control group of regular-admit students entering during this period had a mean score of 613. The special-admit students entering after 1981 had a mean MCAT score (new MCAT) of 9.0; the regular-admit students entering during this period had a mean score of 11.0.
- *Graduation rate.* The special-admit students had a graduation rate of 94 percent; the regular-admit students had a graduation rate of 98 percent. For those students who graduated, the mean time to graduation was the same for both groups (4.2 years).
- *NBME scores.* The mean score for NBME-I was 444 for the special-admit students and 530 for the regular admit students. The mean score for NBME-II was 437 for the special-admit students and 527 for the regular admit students.

- *Residency training.* For both special-admit and regular-admit students, 82 percent of graduates completed their initial choice of residency. Three-fourths of both groups selected primary-care residencies. There was no difference between the two groups in the number of residents who were identified as having academic problems. There was also no difference between the two groups in the number of residents who received special honors, such as being identified as the "best resident" or being selected to be chief resident.

- *Board certification.* 80 percent of special-admit graduates and 85 percent of regular-admit graduates were board-certified in their specialty, a difference that was not found to be statistically significant.

- *Involvement in teaching health professions students.* 51 percent of special-admit graduates and 57 percent of regular-admit graduates reported involvement in teaching health professions students as part of their practice, a difference that was not found to be statistically significant.

- *Professional and personal satisfaction with a medical career.* Both groups of students were satisfied with having chosen medicine as a career, with their current specialty, and with their current practice situation. However, when asked to rate their overall satisfaction with their current life, the special-admit students reported a significantly higher level of personal satisfaction than their regular-admit classmates.

The results of this study by Davidson and Lewis, when combined with the results of the other studies described above, offer a well-supported conclusion about the ultimate effects of the affirmative action programs created to increase the racial and ethnic diversity of the medical profession before many of these programs were prohibited by the Bakke decision. Students admitted under affirmative action programs came to medical school with somewhat lower grades and MCAT scores than their regular-admit classmates. Consistent with the research described in chapter 4, these students also tended to have lower grades early in medical school and lower scores on the licensure examinations. A few more of the special-admit students failed medical school, although the overwhelming majority—well over 90 percent —of both groups graduated successfully. By the time the affirmative action students entered residency training, whatever academic differences they once had were largely dissipated, as reflected in a level of clinical and professional quality that was essentially identical to their classmates admitted under the traditional program.

The decade or so of affirmative action admission that preceded the Bakke decision added substantially to the racial and ethnic diversity of the medical profession, brought a substantial number of new practitioners to underserved communities that were largely poor and minority, and did so without any decrement in clinical skill or professional quality. These conclusions are further supported by the results of a series of smaller studies confirming that many URM students admitted to medical school with lower grades or MCAT scores relative to their classmates were nonetheless fully capable of completing medical school and demonstrating complete clinical competence.[15]

Writing in 1990, Sedlacek and Prieto reviewed the literature available at that time that addressed factors that predicted success in medical school for URM students. They looked both at success in the first two years of medical school and success in the clinical years of medical school, concluding: "First, traditional predictors such as MCAT scores and college GPAs appear to have some validity in predicting the success of minority medical students. Second, nontraditional predictors also appear to have some validity in predicting minority students' success." From their review, they identified a series of noncognitive characteristics, such as positive self-concept, realistic self-appraisal, and successful leadership experience that appeared to predict success in medical school at least as well as MCAT scores and GPAs. They suggested that "minority students' potential cannot be evaluated completely and fairly without measuring noncognitive areas."[16]

Tekian published a similar review of the literature in 1997, coming to similar conclusions: "While these studies have determined that URM students' scores on cognitive tests may be lower than majority students' scores, these students do eventually pass, with little difference in clinical grades. Consequently, many high-risk minority students who are admitted to medical school become excellent physicians."[17]

In 1998 researchers at the AAMC looked at how well MCAT scores predicted outcomes in medical school across racial and ethnic groups, evaluating the scores of more than 12,000 students. Their conclusions only underscore what seems to be the principal conclusion from our consideration of the policy implications of affirmative action programs and other similar programs intended to increase the diversity of the medical profession: "All too often, easily attainable quantitative data, such as test scores and grades, are taken as infallible measures of skill levels. In reality, the best available predictors of achievement do not even approximate perfect prediction."[18]

Efforts to Increase the Diversity of Medical Students after Bakke

While affirmative action programs seem to have been consistently successful in drawing more URM students into the medical profession without a resulting decrement in clinical or professional quality, the constraints on the process with which these programs select students that resulted from the Supreme Court's Bakke decision had a clear impact on the number of URM students entering medical school. As described above, that number remained essentially flat from 1978, the year of the Bakke decision, through the early 1990s. However, the 1990s saw a pattern of increasing numbers of URM medical students, largely the result of a series of programs that targeted URM students but did not use race or ethnicity as the principal selection criterion. These programs were typically of three general types, each of which is discussed below: (1) programs to encourage high school students to consider a health professions career and offering academic support in pursuit of that goal; (2) programs to offer academic enrichment and other types of support to URM college students who are considering a health professions career; and (3) post-baccalaureate programs to offer students who have graduated from college additional instruction and support to encourage and enable their application to medical school.

Programs to Encourage High School Students to Consider a Health Professions Career

The AAMC has focused considerable attention on the issue of increasing the racial and ethnic diversity of students entering medical school. However, that goal still remains problematic, as Anderson reported in 2003 in the AAMC's newsletter: "While gains have been made in encouraging students who are members of underrepresented minority (URM) groups to apply to medical school, the primary reason for minority under-representation in medicine—the limited number of academically well-prepared students with diverse backgrounds in the applicant pool—remains. . . . Critical to ensuring more diversity in medical education are the numerous health sciences professions 'pipeline' programs."[19]

In response to the leveling of the number of URM students entering medical school, in 1991 the AAMC established its "3000 by 2000" program. Supported by medical schools throughout the country, the program "sought to increase the number of underrepresented racial/ethnic minority students matriculating annually in medical school from what was then 1,584 students to 3,000 students by the year 2000."[20] As a core component of this effort, and in collaboration with the Robert Wood Johnson Foundation, the AAMC began its Health Professions Partnership Initiative (HPPI) in 1996.[21] The initiative provided funding for health professions schools and colleges or universities to partner with K–12 school systems to target students from URM or other disadvantaged groups. The program's goals were to help these students improve their academic achievement, encourage them to attend college, and encourage them to consider a health professions career following college.

In 2006 a special issue of the AAMC's journal, *Academic Medicine,* contained a series of reports on the success attained and problems faced by some of the more successful HPPI initiatives. Slater and Iler reported on the partnership between the Mt. Sinai School of Medicine, the City University of New York, and the New York City school system.[22] As part of this initiative, two new magnet schools were opened, one in Queens and one in Manhattan. Each targeted children from grades 6–12; each had an enriched program of science education. In addition, the school in Manhattan, focusing on children from East Harlem, included the participation of residents in internal medicine and pediatrics from Mt. Sinai. While the program had a number of successes, the inability of the New York City school system to provide the needed resources substantially limited both the enrollment in the schools and the success of the program in achieving its goals.

A second HPPI initiative, described by Flores and Dominguez, was launched in 1996 by the University of California, San Francisco's School of Medicine at its branch in Fresno, located in a large agricultural region in California's San Joaquin Valley.[23] Working with local schools, UCSF created a strong academic program within a local high school, focusing on strengthening students' preparation in math and sciences. Referred to as the "Doctors Academy," the program enrolled 255 students over a several-year period. From its first two cohorts completing high school, all of the students graduated from high school and entered a four-year college or university. Based on the success of the Doctors Academy, the program established a second program in a local junior high school, fondly referred to as the "Junior Doctors Academy." Realizing the rigor and resulting academic challenge of its high school program, the Junior Doctors Academy hopes to prepare students for their entry into high school.

Beyond AAMC's HPPI initiative, a number of medical schools throughout the country have created and maintained similar programs targeting students in the precollege years. Among the most successful of these has been the Stanford Medical Youth Science program (SMYSP) at Stanford University. As described by Dr. Marilyn Winkleby, the founder and faculty advisor to SMYSP, the program is "based on the premise that there are large numbers of low-income students who are interested in the health sciences but lack the academic preparation, career-building skills, peer and academic support, and understanding of the college admissions process to succeed in higher education."[24] Since its inception in 1988, SMYSP has brought 20–25 high school students from low-income families to the Stanford campus for a five-week summer residential program, where they receive instruction and direct participation in sciences, direct mentoring by Stanford students, college admissions preparation, and the establishment of a long-term relation with SMYSP staff to assist them in subsequent career counseling. Over the 18 years of the program, 405 students have completed SMYSP, 59 percent of whom were from URM groups. Of these students, 100 percent graduated from high school and 99 percent were admitted to college. Of students admitted to college (and not still in college), 81 percent earned a four-year degree. Of these college graduates, 44 percent either are or are training to become health professionals, including 32 students admitted to medical school. While this record of success seems clear, Winkleby points out that there is no comparison group of similarly qualified students not participating in SMYSP, thus making it difficult to evaluate the actual effect of the program on these students.

A similar program, referred to as the Summer Medical program (SMP), was established in 1972 by the New Jersey Medical School. Targeting high school students from socially or economically disadvantaged families who were college-bound, SMP worked with these students during the summer to provide them "with previews of college science courses and help in developing their noncognitive skills."[25] Between 1972 and 1998, 1,722 high school students were involved in the program. Of the students who have participated in the various programs offered by SMP, 36 percent eventually entered health professions schools. As with the data from Stanford's SMYSP program, these data have no comparison group, so it is difficult to assess accurately the specific effect the program had on the academic and professional paths these students followed.

Bediako and colleagues reported on the success of the Ventures In Education (VIE) program, an independent, nonprofit organization funded by the Josiah Macy Foundation.[26] First established in 1985, VIE provided academic enrichment to economically disadvantaged high school students from several different areas of the country, with an emphasis on strengthening science and math skills in preparation for college and eventually for a health career. Of the 981 graduates of VIE between 1985 and 1989, 136 (13.9%) had taken the MCAT, 109 (11.1%) had applied to medical school, 75 (7.3%) had been accepted, and 72 (7.3%) had entered medical school. Of the 72 students entering medical school, 60 (83%) were from a URM group. Not surprisingly, the 72 students entering medical school had higher grades in high school and higher SAT scores than other students in the program. As with the previous studies, it is difficult to tell from these data the extent to which the program had a direct effect on the career trajectories of the students entering medical school, as there was no comparison group.

Carline, Patterson, and colleagues published two separate reviews of the literature on pre-college enrichment programs targeting minority or other disadvantaged students with the goal of encouraging them to enter a health profession. In 1998 they reviewed 19 different articles describing 27 programs. From this review the authors concluded: "Most evaluations depended on measuring the percentages of program participants who went on to complete college or who entered health-related fields. . . . The lack of comparison groups severely limits the ability to state that program participation significantly contributed to academic success or career choice. . . . Without clarification of how an activity is expected to affect an outcome, evaluation activities are too general to clearly assist in the interpretation of program outcomes."[27]

In 2006, Patterson and Carline again reviewed the available literature on the success of partnerships between health professions schools and public schools in encouraging minority or otherwise disadvantaged students to go to college and enter a health professions school.[28] They concluded that the optimal strategies for such programs focus on general academic enhancement and targeted instructional enhancement in science and math. Echoing the conclusion from their earlier review, they again point to a pattern of apparent success but inadequate outcomes measures to be able to evaluate the actual contributions of these pipeline programs to the ultimate success of their students.

Did these pre-college pipeline programs work? This was the question posed in 2006 by Charles Terrell, the chief diversity officer of the AAMC and the director of the HPPI. Terrell acknowledged that the AAMC's "3000 by 2000" initiative did not meet its goals. Rather than having 3,000 URM students in medical school in the year 2000, there were only 1,700, an increase of fewer than 200 URM students over the period of a decade. Funding for the HPPI initiative expired at the end of 2005.[29] "Did the HPPI projects work?" Terrell asks. He goes on to say, "Unfortunately, we will be joining the long line of researchers and educators saying that little research has been conducted to evaluate the effectiveness of these educational interventions. Without rigorous research and outcomes, it is difficult to determine any program's effectiveness and to identify the specific intervention strategies that were most effective for supporting underrepresented minority students interested in entering the health professions."[30]

It appears that a conclusive answer to the question of efficacy—did the programs actually change the career trajectory of the students they supported, or did they rather simply serve to support the strongest students who were headed to health professions schools anyway?—will need to await more carefully thought out research and evaluation methodologies. We do, however, have some data about those students for whom the programs did *not* work. In 1999 Thurmond and Cregler reported on the results of their survey of 123 students who, between 1984 and 1991, had completed the Student Educational Enrichment Program, a high school "pipeline" program operated since 1978 by the Medical College of Georgia. Of the students they surveyed, 96 percent indicated that, at the time they participated in the program as high school students, they had hoped to be physicians. While nearly all attended college, only 26 of the 123 (21%) students had attended or were attending medical school. When the researchers asked those students who had not attended medical school why they had changed their minds, two of the principal responses were "fear of problems with grades" and "feeling of inadequate preparation in science (chemistry most frequently cited)."[31]

The numerous "pipeline" programs created throughout the decades following the Bakke decision have had substantial success in getting talented but disadvantaged high school students into the health professions pipeline and into college. However, for many of these students that pipeline leaks badly somewhere during the college experience. As Thurmond and Cregler concluded, a major contributor to that leakage is inadequate preparation of students for the rigors of the college chemistry classroom, the first step toward entry to medical school. These authors suggest that in order to stem this leakage "public schools, colleges, and medical schools need to work in concert to reach students interested in medicine early for extra courses in chemistry and other basic sciences."[32]

As described in chapter 1, the premedical pipeline continues to leak badly, even at highly competitive universities such as Stanford and the University of California, Berkeley. It is not clear, however, that the appropriate solution is to give disadvantaged high school students more instruction in chemistry. Such an approach takes as given the pedagogical approach and curricular content of college chemistry courses, assuming that if problems develop, they lie with the students.

Programs to Offer Support to URM College Students

Beyond encouraging more URM students to consider a health career while they are still in high school, a range of programs have been created by universities and professional schools that instead target URM students who are already in college. I describe three of the most long-standing and successful of these below.

HEALTH CAREERS OPPORTUNITY PROGRAM (HCOP)

In 1972 the federal government established Health Careers Opportunity Program (HCOP) with the goal of "increas[ing] the number of individuals from disadvantaged backgrounds in the health and allied health professions." By "disadvantaged backgrounds" the government meant "from an environment that has inhibited the individual from obtaining the knowledge, skills, and abilities to succeed in a health profession . . . and/or a student from a family with an annual income below a level based on low-income thresholds according to family size."[33] By focusing on students from low-income families or educationally disadvantaged backgrounds, the program had the goal of increasing the racial and ethnic diversity of the medical profession and other health professions without specifically focusing on race. Because URM students are statistically more likely to come from such a disadvantaged background, programs targeting disadvantaged students generally will likely be more racially and ethnically diverse than the general population of medical school applicants. While HCOP has included pipeline programs focusing on K–12 education, many of the programs have specifically targeted students in college. For the programs funded during fiscal years 2004 and 2005, about two-thirds of the nearly 24,000 students participating in HCOP programs were in colleges or universities. HCOP programs often included recruiting disadvantaged college students into a health professions pathway as well as supporting those students already in such a career path. Programs used strategies such as offering counseling and mentoring, strengthening students' academic preparation, offering students research opportunities, and exposing students to community-based primary health care settings.

CENTERS OF EXCELLENCE PROGRAMS (COE)

Centers of Excellence (COE) was created by Congress in 1988 with the goal of "strengthen[ing] the national capacity to train students from minority groups that are under-represented in the health professions and build a more diverse health care workforce."[34] It targets medical, dental, and other health professions schools that typically enroll a higher percentage of URM students than the national average. The program also explicitly includes certain historically black colleges and universities. A principal focus of the program is for health professions schools to work with preprofessional undergraduate students to enhance their academic performance so as to create a more competitive applicant pool. The program supports schools in efforts to address minority health issues, to foster both faculty and student research in this area, and to support community-based clinical training.

MINORITY MEDICAL EDUCATION PROGRAM (MMEP)/
SUMMER MEDICAL AND DENTAL EDUCATION PROGRAM (SMDEP)

Responding to the dampening effect the Bakke decision had on the enrollment of URM students in medical schools, in 1988 the Robert Wood Johnson Foundation (RWJF) established the Minority Medical Education Program (MMEP). Its purpose was to "provide a summer enrichment experience for minority college students who possess the academic qualifications that would gain entrance to medical school."[35] As described by Bergeisen and Cantor, "The purpose of the program was not to expand the overall applicant pool but, rather, to increase the acceptance rates of those individuals with the requisite credentials."[36] To achieve this goal, MMEP focused on the development of summer enrichment programs for URM college students who already were interested in applying to medical school and who had an academic record that appeared to make them competitive for medical school. It offered these students academic enrichment in biology, chemistry, and physics; help in preparing for the MCAT; and mentoring and counseling support to assist students with the process of applying to medical school. From its inception, MMEP was designed, not as a remedial education program, helping students who had had difficulty in the premedical sciences, but rather as an enrichment program, helping students who had previously demonstrated success in the sciences to become more competitive applicants. Thus MMEP was not strictly designed as a "pipeline" program intended to increase the number of URM students interested in medical school or other health professions schools.

Responding to the success of MMEP, in 2003 the RWJF expanded and extended the program to include premedical students who were economically, socially, or educationally disadvantaged. In 2005 the program was further extended to include students interested in becoming dentists and was renamed as the Summer Medical and Dental Education Program (SMDEP).

A crucial issue for medical educators has been to get some assessment, using valid indicators of outcomes, of the success of the programs described above. To this end, the results of two research studies evaluating these programs were published in 1998. Cantor and colleagues reported their study of the effectiveness of the MMEP in increasing the chances of its participants being accepted to medical school.[37] (Recall that all MMEP participants had previously identified medicine as their career goal.) The researchers looked at all URM applicants to medical schools in the 1997 application cohort. Of 3,830 URM applicants nationally, 452 had participated in an MMEP summer program. The rate of acceptance to medical school for the MMEP participants was 49.3 percent, compared to 41.6 percent for non-participants. Since MMEP participants were selected from among those students with the highest undergraduate grades, the authors evaluated the effect of program participation in a multivariate format, controlling for grades, test scores, and demographic variables. Controlling for these factors, the odds of MMEP participants gaining acceptance to medical school were greater than those of non-participants.

While Cantor and colleagues looked specifically at one admissions cohort of the MMEP program, Carline and colleagues took a somewhat broader view, reporting their review of all published studies evaluating enrichment programs that had the goal of increasing the number of URM students entering medicine. They were able to identify eighteen articles published between 1966 and 1996 that reported on the outcomes of enrichment programs targeting URM college students. A number of these programs received funding from HCOP, described above. The strategies most commonly used by these programs included academic enhancement, admission preparation, and mentoring. The outcome most frequently reported was, "the percentage of participants that subsequently entered medical schools." Most of the programs reported acceptance rates in the 70–80 percent range, suggesting a high level of success. However, the authors also underscored an important finding: "While the medical school matriculation rate was quite high, these results were difficult to interpret as the studies did not use control groups. The evaluations could not demonstrate, therefore, that the programs were responsible for increased admission of minorities to medical schools. . . . Without this type of public discussion, enrichment programs for underrepresented minorities may continue to appear to be worthwhile endeavors, but lacking solid support and foundation and vulnerable to losing funding."[38]

Without clear evidence that the programs actually increased the number of URM students applying to and accepted by medical school, it is difficult to know how much value was returned by the financial investment in them. It is entirely possible that program participants had a high level of medical school acceptances, not because the programs added to the "pipeline" of URM students interested in a medical career, but rather because they selected as participants students who brought with them levels of academic attainment and personal strengths that made it more likely they would be accepted to medical school. That these programs are vulnerable to losing funding based on the weakness of the evidence showing that they increased the pipeline of qualified applicants was reflected in the fact that between Fiscal Year 2004 and Fiscal Year 2008 federal funding for COE was cut from $33.7 million to $12.8 million,[39] and funding for HCOP was cut from $36.2 million to $9.8 million.[40]

Post-baccalaureate Premedical Programs

Not every student who hopes to attend medical school is successful in gaining admission, despite having completed the premedical requirements as an undergraduate. Weak or incomplete training in the premedical sciences may make a student less competitive for a coveted medical school slot and result in rejection rather than admission. For such students who have graduated from college yet who still hope to attend medical school, a number of colleges and universities have organized formal programs that provide additional training in the premedical sciences as well as mentorship and support (e.g., MCAT test preparation). Referred to as post-baccalaureate premedical programs (PBPM), they assist students in completing or strengthening their premedical science preparation and in becoming more familiar with the process of applying to medical school. In 2008 a Web site maintained by the AAMC listed more than 100 such programs.[41]

Different PBPM programs focus on different target groups. Some look for students who have had a strong academic record but who came to the decision to apply to medical school later in the process. Such students simply need the coursework they are missing plus general assistance with the application process. One such program is at Bryn Mawr College, a highly selective women's college in Pennsylvania. Bryn Mawr's program, founded in 1972, is described as "designed for women and men like you who are highly motivated to pursue a career in medicine but have not taken the required premedical courses as undergraduates. . . . We are highly selective and typically accept no more than 75 women and men per year."[42] Given the highly competitive nature of the students selected for Bryn Mawr's program, it is not surprising that they report a greater than 98 percent success rate for their students' gaining admission to medical school.

In contrast to Bryn Mawr's program, the seven PBPM programs offered by the University of California's medical schools have the specific mission of, "increas[ing] the number of physicians who practice in shortage areas of California, by assisting capable and dedicated students from disadvantaged backgrounds in gaining admission to medical school."[43] To this end, many of the PBPM programs offered by the University of California focus on applicants who have previously applied to medical school but were not accepted by any school. Many of the applicants to these programs have a relatively weak academic record in the premedical sciences and need to strengthen their scientific knowledge and their preparation for the MCAT.

One of the first PBPM programs in the country was established in 1969 at Wayne State University School of Medicine. The program was designed with a specific focus on African American students who had applied to medical school but had been rejected.[44] As part of the pre-Bakke affirmative action era, the Wayne State program brought between five and ten African American students to campus for an intensive ten-month program that helped them to strengthen their science preparation, their overall academic skills, and their personal commitment to a career as a physician. The program was structured such that every student who maintained a B average throughout the program was guaranteed admission to the Wayne State School of Medicine. After the Bakke decision in 1978, the program shifted its focus to disadvantaged students without specific regard to race or ethnicity.

Between 1969 and 1992, 192 of 214 African American students (90%) admitted to the program successfully completed it and entered medical school; 160 of the 192 medical school matriculants (83%) completed medical school. Of the 58 non-African American disadvantaged students admitted after the Bakke decision, 54 (93%) entered medical school and 51 (94%) completed medical school. The program has contributed substantially to the professional success of hundreds of disadvantaged students who otherwise would not have had the opportunity to attend medical school. The university continues to offer a PBPM program, maintaining its focus on "disadvantaged medical school applicants from Michigan who have been denied admission, but who appear to have the potential for academic success."[45]

In the early years of the Wayne State program, a number of students who had done well in the PBPM science courses still had difficulty in the first-year biochemistry course in the medical school. As described by the program's administrator, "When students who had successfully completed the postbaccalaureate program nonetheless did not perform well in the medical school's first-year biochemistry course, the university's survey courses in inorganic chemistry and biochemistry were analyzed. This analysis revealed that in each course some covered material had little value in preparing students for the medical school's biochemistry course. Thereafter, better focused inorganic chemistry and biochemistry courses were developed and taught by medical school faculty."[46]

The program's response to the problems students encountered in the medical school's biochemistry course holds particular relevance for our discussion of the optimal pedagogy of premedical science courses. Recognizing that a student's lack of success may reflect a combination of academic weakness on the part of the student and pedagogical weakness on the part of the university, the program was able to increase students' success by focusing simultaneously on both.

The School of Medicine at Southern Illinois University at Carbondale (SIU) was founded in 1970 and accepted its first entering class in 1972. In addition to its standard medical curriculum, SIU also offered a special program titled the Medical Education Preparatory Program, referred to by its acronym MEDPREP. From its inception, MEDPREP had as its goals to "train . . . primary care physicians who would establish rural and inner-city practices" and to "assist minority medical students and other students with disadvantaged backgrounds to prepare for admission and success in medical school."[47] As described on its Web site, "MEDPREP was designed as a two-year postbaccalaureate program for disadvantaged students. It provides an environment in which students can hone their test-taking skills and enhance their academic record before matriculating in a health professional school."[48] In order to be eligible for the program, an applicant must be from an educationally or economically disadvantaged background and must have completed all or most of the math and science prerequisites for medical school with a grade of C or above. MEDPREP defines as "science prerequisites" two years of chemistry with lab, two years of biology, and one year of physics with lab. The program targets students who meet these requirements who are not currently competitive for medical school admission. Those students accepted into the program complete a two-year post-baccalaureate curriculum. The first year provides additional instruction in chemistry, biology, and physics as well as courses to improve general verbal and learning skills. The second year, during which students apply to medical school, incorporates enrichment courses and additional science courses intended to prepare the student for the first year of medical school.

In its more than 30 years of existence, MEDPREP has enrolled over 1,000 students, more than three-fourths of which are from URM groups. Sixty-three percent of its graduates have successfully enrolled in medical school, with an additional 5 percent enrolling in other health professions schools. Of its students accepted to a health professions school, 87 percent have graduated.[49] A study of students graduating from MEDPREP in the period 1972–1992 found that, of those students achieving board certification in a medical specialty, 70 percent were certified in a primary care specialty.[50] Even though there is no comparison group by which to evaluate these outcomes, it nonetheless appears that MEDPREP has attained its dual goals of training more primary care physicians and increasing the diversity of the medical profession.

The University of California at Davis (UCD) established its PBPM program in 1991, targeting students from educationally, socially, or economically disadvantaged backgrounds who had previously applied to medical school but failed to gain acceptance. The program acknowledged that "although grades and test scores have some relevancy, they are not nor should they be the sole indicators of an applicant's success in the program or in medical school."[51] Accordingly, the program considered grades and MCAT scores but also looked at a student's motivation, personal background, previous experience, and potential for practicing in an underserved community in California. In addition, the program looked carefully for possible explanations and appropriate solutions for a student's previously weak academic performance.

Unlike the Wayne State program, in which all students who meet certain academic goals are guaranteed admission to medical school, the UCD program helps its students prepare for re-application to medical school but does not guarantee admission. The program has had considerable success in placing its students in medical school, with 95 of 115 participating students (83%) having gained acceptance to major medical schools in the United States.

Cognizant of the previous criticism of early pipeline programs and college enrichment programs—that the programs had no comparison group to validate the actual effect of the program on students' success—Grumbach and Chen undertook a study of five separate PBPM programs operated by University of California medical schools, one of which was at UCD.[52] They evaluated the outcomes for 265 participants in these programs, comparing their success in gaining admission to medical school to that of 396 college graduates who had applied to one of these programs but not been accepted. They found that 67.6 percent of PBPM participants gained admission to medical school, while only 22.5 percent of non-participants gained admission, leading them to conclude, "Postbaccalaureate premedical programs appear to be an effective intervention to increase the number of medical school matriculants for disadvantaged and underrepresented groups."[53]

Will students who have experienced academic weakness in the traditional premedical sciences and who then go on to take additional science courses after graduation be able to be successful in medical school? This question is of course crucial in evaluating PBPM programs as a means to increase the diversity of the medical profession. Hojat and colleagues looked at students entering Jefferson Medical College between 1985 and 1987, comparing 133 students who had taken some form of extra preparation in the sciences with 463 students who had not taken extra work.[54] They found that the students electing to take extra courses following graduation had lower grades, both as undergraduates and in the first two years of medical school.

Most of the students in the Hojat study had taken the extra post-baccalaureate science courses on their own, not in a formally structured PBPM program. Giordani and colleagues looked at the success of 15 URM medical students at the University of Michigan who had completed the university's formal PBPM program, comparing their success with 48 other medical students who had taken independent post-baccalaureate science courses and with 443 medical students who had only the traditional premedical science courses. The students from the formal PBPM program had lower undergraduate GPAs (both science and non-science) and lower MCAT scores than either the traditional students or the students with independent post-baccalaureate work. Despite these differences, there were no significant differences in their performance in the first year of medical school, with most of the PBPM students scoring close to the class mean.[55]

Interestingly, while undergraduate grades and MCAT scores predicted first-year grades for the traditional students, these predictors of early medical school success had no significant association with the first-year scores of the PBPM students. Despite what looks initially like a substantially weaker undergraduate preparation for medical school, the PBPM students "perform with little difference in academic achievement and have the potential to become excellent physicians."[56]

These results again call into question the assumption that weak academic performance in premedical sciences is principally a reflection on the student. That many of these students, often coming from disadvantaged backgrounds, can succeed in an appropriately structured PBPM program, and subsequently in medical school, suggests that the pedagogy of premedical science education is every bit as much a factor in the students' early academic difficulties as is the student's inherent academic abilities. In a series of interviews with URM students from a disadvantaged background who were selected for a PBPM program, Frohna confirmed that, given positive attitudes, realistic self-assessment, and clear personal commitment, these students can be fully successful when offered science preparation in an appropriately structured pedagogy.[57]

Connecting Research on Diversity to Research on Professional Outcomes

For the four decades between 1968 and 2008, a variety of programs were put into place nationally, with one consistent goal: to increase the racial and ethnic diversity of students entering medical school, and ultimately of the medical profession. During the first ten years of this period, the principle focus was on affirmative action programs that explicitly targeted students from URM groups. When in 1978 the Supreme Court's Bakke decision prohibited explicit racial or ethnic preferences, the programs broadened their focus to include students from a range of disadvantaged backgrounds, including social, educational, and economic disadvantage.

The effort to get more students from disadvantaged backgrounds into medical school included three principal thrusts: increasing the pipeline of students entering college with the goal of entering medicine or another a health profession, strengthening and enriching the experience of disadvantaged students in four-year colleges or universities so as to make them more competitive in the medical school application process, and offering formally structured post-baccalaureate education to strengthen the premedical preparation of disadvantaged students who had not been successful in gaining entry to medical school.

The associations between undergraduate science performance and subsequent performance in medical school identified in chapter 4 are quite consistent with the outcomes of the research evaluating the impact of affirmative action admissions, both the pre-Bakke programs that explicitly targeted URM groups and the post-Bakke programs that targeted disadvantaged students more broadly. Programs that offer admission to students with lower premedical grades and MCAT scores report that these students often score somewhat lower in their early medical school classes and their initial licensure examination (NBME I or USMLE I). However, the vast majority—typically substantially more than 90 percent—of students admitted to medical school under the various special admissions considerations successfully completed the first two years of medical school and moved on to their clinical training.

Once in their clinical training, we again see a pattern that is consistent with the research summarized in chapter 4. Performance in the first two years of medical school has little association with performance in a clinical context. Whether measured as evaluations by clerkship directors, reports of residency directors, or national licensure exams that test clinical skills, students admitted under special considerations and students admitted under traditional review methods become largely indistinguishable as clinicians, and the quality of the professional practice of the two groups is essentially the same. There simply is no evidence that four decades of special admissions programs targeting students from disadvantaged backgrounds has had an adverse effect on the clinical or professional quality of the physicians trained through these programs.

While there is no evidence of a quality decrement resulting from special admissions programs, there is evidence of one effect that is worth noting, especially in the context of the medical manpower needs of the twenty-first century. Students admitted under the special consideration programs were significantly more likely to select a primary care profession, to locate their practice in medical manpower shortage areas, and to provide care to low-income or poor patients. Especially in states such as California, where assuring adequate medical manpower for an increasingly diverse population is a state policy priority, the positive impact of affirmative action and other diversity enhancement programs holds particular relevance.

Given the positive effect that the special admissions programs have had without a corresponding decrement in clinical quality, we should ask whether the various pipeline programs described above have been a major contributor to the success we have had in training a more diverse medical profession. Here it is difficult to give a reliable answer. While it certainly appears that the various programs working with high school students or enriching the college experience of premedical students have had a positive effect on the number of qualified students applying to medical school, the research that documents this success in a reliable and valid manner is largely missing. Usually due to the lack of a comparison group in the analysis of program outcomes, it has not been possible to determine whether program activities or preselection bias accounted for the high rates of reported success. Future research on these types of programs must keep this issue always in mind.

Finally, research presented in this chapter has underscored a concern identified in chapter 1. As described above, Thurmond and Cregler surveyed minority college students identified as gifted in high school who had participated in a pipeline enrichment program but nonetheless had dropped out of premedical studies. When asked why they had lost their interest in becoming a physician, these students cited low grades and bad experiences in their early premedical science courses, principally chemistry.[58] The very same explanation was given by the students we interviewed at Stanford University and the University of California, Berkeley. Those students from disadvantaged backgrounds who successfully complete the premedical science curriculum, even if they do not do as well as students toward the top of the distribution, will almost certainly be successful in medical school. However, substantial numbers of other students, most of whom are just as talented as those who persist and succeed in entering medical school, never submit an application to medical school. Their early college experience in chemistry and other premedical sciences has convinced them, rightly or wrongly, that dropping out of the premedical pipeline was the appropriate thing to do. In thinking about how best to organize the teaching of premedical science, we must always keep these students in mind and seek to find ways to stem this unnecessary leakage of otherwise qualified students.

Nontraditional Programs of Medical Education and Their Success in Training Qualified Physicians

Since approximately 1925, the vast majority of medical schools in the United States have relied on a single paradigm for the selection of new students from among those submitting applications. Candidates were evaluated primarily based on their academic achievement in the standardized premedical curriculum of chemistry, biology, and physics. That course sequence, first proposed in the late 1800s by educators such as Daniel Coit Gilman of Johns Hopkins and Charles W. Eliot of Harvard and first standardized by the Council on Medical Education between 1905 and 1914, became the norm for most schools. In many states, including California and New York, it was also the law. Medical schools also incorporated, to varying degrees, assessment of a candidate's noncognitive strengths through personal interviews and written materials included in the application. However, for most of the last century an applicant's performance in the premedical sciences predominated in the selection process.

I refer to a "paradigm of selection" for two reasons. A paradigm has at least two aspects: (1) it reflects a dominant model of organization or action, and (2) it represents a generally accepted view or perspective underlying the practice of a science or a discipline.[1] The widespread adoption of a standardized model of the premedical science curriculum occurred nearly a century ago. Victor C. Vaughan described this model in 1914 in his address to the Council on Medical Education (CME): "No man is fit to study medicine, unless he is acquainted, and pretty thoroughly acquainted, with the fundamental facts in physical, chemical, and biological subjects."[2] By the mid-1920s, nearly every medical school in the United States had adopted Vaughan's model of the premedical sciences required of entering students. In 2008 more than 90 percent of U.S. medical schools continued to do so.[3]

Premedical education requirements that are based on this model also reflect a dominant way of thinking—a particular view of what underlies medical science that came to be generally accepted. Again, as described by Victor C. Vaughan in 1914, "The facts of the biological, physical, and chemical sciences are the pabulum on which medicine feeds. Without these sciences, everything that goes under the name of medicine is fraud, sham and superstition."[4] Vaughan's words echoed those of Abraham Flexner from his 1910 Report: "The normal rhythm of physiologic function must then remain a riddle to students who cannot think and speak in biological, chemical, and physical language."[5]

Vaughan, Flexner, and other medical educators from that era were in essence arguing two points: (1) medical schools should standardize their premedical entrance requirements to fit the chemistry-biology-physics model; and (2) it is impossible for anyone lacking early training in these sciences to become fully competent as a physician. Based on the belief that science is an absolute prerequisite for clinical competence, Flexner (and the CME before him) used the science-based standards of admission as one of the principal metrics with which he evaluated medical schools as part of his national study. Any school failing to establish and enforce the requirement of college-level courses in chemistry, biology, and physics for admission would, by definition, fail to meet the standards of quality set by the CME and would therefore not get a passing mark. Arguing in a tight tautological circle, Flexner defined "high quality" as having a premedical curriculum centered on chemistry-biology-physics and then defined as "lacking in quality" any medical school that failed to apply such a standard of admission.

Compare the comments of Vaughan and Flexner to those of Drs. Higgins and Reed made in 2007 and cited in chapter 1. Defending the continued role of chemistry and physics as anchors of premedical education, they argued that "these disciplines contribute a great deal to providing the framework for understanding basic principles of medicine."[6] As part of any contemporary discussion of the appropriateness of the current premedical curriculum, many voices will be raised in support of the beliefs voiced by Vaughan, Flexner, Higgins, and Reed. Such beliefs hold that modern medicine, both medical knowledge and medical practice, is built specifically on a foundation of chemistry, biology, and physics and that the absence of these sciences will necessarily call into question the clinical and professional quality of any physician who lacks such a foundation.

Not all medical schools have adopted this dominant model of premedical education, however. We will examine several schools that have stepped outside this premedical paradigm to differing degrees and look for evidence of how the clinical and professional quality of their graduates compares to the quality of graduates selected under the dominant paradigm.

Schools Accepting High School Students into the Study of Medicine

Recall from our discussion in chapters 2 and 3 that the current model of medical education in the United States evolved as an adaptation of the model of medical education that predominated in Europe in the late nineteenth and early twentieth centuries. That model was described extensively as part of the 1932 *Final Report of the Commission on Medical Education.*[7] Students completing their secondary school education who excelled on national examinations such as the *Abitur* in Germany and the *Baccalaureate* in France were then accepted into the medical curriculum of a university. Over a period typically lasting six to seven years, the student would take general arts and humanities courses as well as the science and clinical courses necessary to complete the medical curriculum. There was no distinction made between "premedical" and "medical" courses. Those students who successfully completed the curriculum graduated with their medical degrees. It was only in the United States that educators chose to break this curriculum into two stages: the undergraduate premedical course, which included the sciences of chemistry, biology, and physics; and the medical course, which built on these scientific subjects with courses in physiology, biochemistry, and anatomy, followed by training in a clinical context.

In 1973, the City of New York faced the same problems as other areas of the country in providing for its future medical manpower needs. For New York, there were two principal issues: (1) training enough doctors in the crucial primary care areas of family practice, general internal medicine, and pediatrics to meet the medical needs of New York, especially its urban areas identified as medical manpower shortage areas; and (2) consistent with other areas of the country, making medical education more available to students from underrepresented minority (URM) racial and ethnic groups. To address both issues, in 1973 the City University of New York founded the Sophie Davis School of Biomedical Education located at the City College of New York.[8] Roman and McGanney have described the philosophy behind Sophie Davis:

> In retrospect, two assumptions were apparent in the planning of [Sophie Davis]. First, it was assumed that an alternative pathway to medicine could increase the chances of talented minority and educationally disadvantaged inner-city youths to overcome the premedical studies "screening" effect of the traditional pathway to medicine. . . . [E]vidence has shown that difficulty with introductory science courses causes many minority students to drop out of the medical school pipeline. We at Sophie Davis proposed that courses traditionally taught in the preclinical

years of medical school could be successfully integrated with baccalaureate education without diminishing the quality of the preparation of future physicians.[9]

This statement of the underlying philosophy of Sophie Davis offers a ringing endorsement of the historical European model of medical education, in which talented students coming out of high school are selected for an integrated baccalaureate/medical curriculum. It also underscores a principal thesis of this book—that the classical paradigm of premedical education, especially the introductory science courses, act to "screen" or "weed out" students based on their performance in these courses and that the students screened or weeded out in this manner tend disproportionately to be students from disadvantaged social or educational backgrounds.

The statement of the second philosophical principal underlying Sophie Davis adds additional perspective to our discussion:

Second, it was assumed that the early introduction of a clearly defined institutional mission and an enriched exposure to the social and community health sciences, reinforced with community-based fieldwork experience, could motivate and encourage students to pursue primary care specialties even in the absence of a complementary clinical curriculum.[10]

This statement of the institutional mission of Sophie Davis, based on education in and an understanding of relevant social and community health sciences in addition to the premedical sciences, further differentiates Sophie Davis from the dominant premedical paradigm. Although premedical students have for several decades been encouraged to seek a broad liberal arts education while also completing the required courses in chemistry, biology, and physics, few medical schools have equated the importance of courses in the relevant social sciences with the importance of the natural sciences.

Students at Sophie Davis are selected out of high school using the following criteria: "high-school grade-point averages, the New York State Regents Examination scores, American College Test (ACT) scores, Scholastic Aptitude Test (SAT) scores, personal statement and writing sample, high-school references, extracurricular and community activities, and two interviews."[11] Of the approximately 70 students admitted each year, most come from one of the five boroughs of New York City, with others coming from nearby counties.

Once in Sophie Davis, students take a five-year curriculum at City College of New York that encompasses both a liberal arts curriculum and the social and natural science courses considered to be part of the medical curriculum. Students are required to maintain a minimum grade point average while at City College and, upon completion of the five-year curriculum, to pass Part I of the USMLE exam. Students who meet both these requirements are then assured a clinical training slot in one of several collaborating medical schools in the New York area. The medical degree is granted by the school at which a student receives his or her clinical training.

Of the students who enter Sophie Davis coming out of high school, 82–85 percent successfully complete the program and transfer to another medical school for clinical training.[12] Of 1,400 students graduating from the program between 1973 and 2004, more than 99 percent successfully completed their MD degree at one of the collaborating schools. Of these students, 6 percent were elected to Alpha Omega Alpha, the national medical honor society. Between 1999 and 2003, 83 percent of graduates entered primary care residencies. Data from the study by Roman and McGanney indicate that 65 percent of those graduating between 1977 and 1987 were practicing primary care medicine. Of those graduating between 1977 and 1990, 13 percent were on medical school faculties.[13]

It seems apparent that Sophie Davis has been successful in attaining the two goals it set in 1973 when it was established: it has trained and continues to train substantial numbers of New York students who faced educational or social disadvantages upon completing high school; it has trained substantial numbers of primary care physicians who are now providing care to under-served areas of New York City and State. As summarized by Roman, "The Sophie Davis model suggests that those students who excel in mastering even average complexities of precollegiate sciences can rise to the challenge of our school's rigorous medical school biomedical and sociomedical science curriculum when appropriate academic and personal supports are offered."[14]

The Sophie Davis school is not, of course, the only U.S. medical school that has combined, in one manner or another, the undergraduate baccalaureate curriculum with the medical curriculum. Others have operated successfully for decades.[15] In a review published in 1992, Norman and Calkins identified such programs at 28 medical schools.[16] In 2008, the AAMC identified 44 such programs,[17] one of which is at the Baylor College of Medicine.

As reported by Thomson and colleagues, in 1994 Baylor College of Medicine and the University of Texas-Pan American jointly established their Premedical Honors College (PHC).[18] PHC targets a 13-county region of South Texas in which the population is 82 percent Hispanic and which for some time has been a medically underserved area. By selecting qualified high school students from this area and providing them with combined baccalaureate and medical training, the program has the dual goals of increasing the availability of primary care services and increasing the racial and ethnic diversity of the medical profession in Texas. The program selects high school students from this geographic area based on their academic performance in high school, their SAT scores, letters of recommendation, and an assessment of noncognitive characteristics such as maturity, life experiences, motivation, personality, and communication skills. Students are expected to take traditional undergraduate courses in chemistry and biology. They also work in local hospitals and clinics to become familiar with the process of health care delivery and with the health problems and conditions confronting the local population. If they maintain a minimum level of academic performance in these undergraduate activities, the students are then guaranteed a place in the Baylor medical school.

At the time of the report by Thomson and colleagues, 71 students had completed the undergraduate portion of the curriculum, 84.5 percent of whom had successfully matriculated at the Baylor College of Medicine. All of the students who did not enter medical school enrolled in another graduate or professional program in a health-related field. Comparing PHC students with other college students from similar social and educational backgrounds, the odds of a PHC student matriculating to medical school were seven times higher than for a non-PHC student. As with Sophie Davis, PHC has succeeded by identifying fully qualified high school students who come from otherwise disadvantaged social and educational backgrounds. As we have documented at both Stanford University and the University of California Berkeley (see chapter 1), and as has been the case at many other colleges and universities, these students typically face immense challenges when they enroll in the traditional premedical curriculum at a large college or university with the result that many leave the premedical pipeline and never submit an application to a medical school. Schools such as PHC and Sophie Davis present an eminently reasonable alternative for these students, with no evidence that students who successfully complete the curriculum are lacking in any aspect of clinical or professional quality.

Medical Schools That Accept Students Early in Their Undergraduate Experience

In 1920, two years of undergraduate study in an approved college or university was the norm for admission to most U.S. medical schools. By the 1950s that norm had grown to four years, where it remains today. A substantial majority of students applying to medical school do so after having completed a four-year undergraduate program; however, a few schools have elected to evaluate and admit students before those students have completed their undergraduate curriculum.

In 1983 Boston University School of Medicine (BUSM) established such a program in its Early Medical School Selection Program (EMSSP). As described by

Edelin and Ugbolue, EMSSP was established with the goal of increasing the enrollment of URM students and other disadvantaged students in medical school.[19] It is
a partnership between BUSM and 13 different colleges and universities, each of
which has substantial URM enrollment among its undergraduates. Students from
these institutions are eligible to apply to BUSM after they have completed their
sophomore year of undergraduate study. Admissions evaluation involves a combination of high school grades, college grades, SAT scores, letters of recommendation,
an admissions essay, and an interview. Those students accepted into the program
spend the summer before their junior year at BUSM, returning to their home institution for their junior year. They then spend their senior year at BUSM, completing the requirements for their bachelor's degree and taking science courses such as
biochemistry and histology as a transition into medical school. All these courses are
credited to the student's bachelor's degree requirements at his or her undergraduate
institution. Students who maintain a minimum grade average, obtain their bachelor's degree from their home institution, and perform adequately on the MCAT (no
minimum score is specified) are then accepted as entering medical students at
BUSM. Since its inception, approximately 60 percent of students admitted to
EMSSP have successfully enrolled at BUSM.

The Mount Sinai School of Medicine in New York City also has a program that
accepts students early in their undergraduate career, although with a focus that differs substantially from that of EMSSP. As discussed in chapter 5, in 1984 the Association of American Medical Colleges issued Physicians for the Twenty-First
Century, reporting the findings of its Project Panel on the General Professional Education of the Physician and College Preparation for Medicine.[20] The report was
intended as a follow-up to the 1932 Commission on Medical Education report,
which had cautioned against "the tendency of medical schools and regulatory bodies to define in detail the range and character of premedical preparation." It argued
instead that "a sound general education is of more value to students of medicine
than a narrow technical training in the premedical sciences."[21]

The AAMC's 1984 report reiterated this concern: "We perceive a continuing erosion of general education for physicians, an erosion that has not been arrested but is
instead accelerating." The report contained specific recommendations for how medical schools should respond to this "continuing erosion" of the quality of the general education that physicians obtain as undergraduates: "In framing criteria for admission to medical school, faculties should require only essential courses. Whenever
possible, these should be part of the core courses that all college students must take.
The practice of medical school admissions committees recommending additional
courses beyond those required for admission should cease. *Some institutions may*

wish to experiment by not recommending any specific course requirement" (emphasis added).[22]

Responding to this admonishment to try something different in the way medical students are selected, in 1989 Mount Sinai School of Medicine initiated its Humanities and Medicine Program (HMP). As explained on its Web site, the program "provides a path to medical school that offers maximum flexibility in the undergraduate years for students to explore their interests in humanities and social sciences at top liberal arts colleges and research universities."[23] Rather than focusing on students from disadvantaged backgrounds, HMP targets some of the top students nationally who are enrolled at highly selective institutions. Students apply to the program during the first semester of their sophomore year of college. Students are selected for admission based on a personal essay, high school and college grades, SAT scores, letters of recommendation, and personal interviews. Those students who are selected for HMP must choose an undergraduate major in the humanities or social sciences (i.e., *not* in the natural sciences); limit their undergraduate science courses to one year of biology and one year of chemistry and attain a grade of B or better in these courses; and attend an eight-week course at MSSM in the summer after their junior year of college, in which they take an abbreviated course that covers organic chemistry and physics, but only those principles of these sciences that have direct relevance to medicine. During this eight-week summer course, students also gain an initial exposure to clinical activities.

Students in HMP enter medical school with an undergraduate education that is substantially more broad-based than most medical students. They also, however, enter with an education in the premedical sciences that is more narrow than most other medical students. This brings up the inevitable questions: How will HMP students do in medical school as compared to their classmates whose premedical education followed the chemistry-biology-physics paradigm? Equally important, what kind of doctors do HMP students become?

These questions were addressed by Rifkin and colleagues in a report published in 2000, comparing the medical school experiences of 85 HMP students with matched cohorts of students with a traditional premedical education. The authors found that

- HMP students were more likely to fail one or more course in the first two years of medical school, with biochemistry being the course most often failed.
- HMP students were more likely to fail the USMLE-I examination on their first try, although all HMP students did eventually pass the exam (it was

noted that all HMP students who failed USMLE-I had a verbal SAT score of
≤ 650).

- There were no significant differences in either the rate of failure in the clinical clerkships or in the rate of attaining honors in the clinical clerkships.

- HMP students were over-represented in those students receiving awards for community service and those students taking leadership positions in student organizations.

- HMP students were more likely than non-HMP students to receive a graduation award upon completing medical school.[24]

Based on these data, Rifkin and colleagues identified two fundamental principles regarding premedical education: (1) "Our experience shows that although students in this program have more academic difficulties in the preclinical years, they excel in the clinical/community setting and have greatly enriched the medical school environment. This program demonstrates that success in medical school does not depend on a traditional premed science curriculum"; and (2) "The Humanities and Medicine Program challenges the long-standing belief that there is a necessary relationship between undergraduate science preparation and the successful completion of medical school and physician excellence."[25]

McMaster University—Further Challenging the Paradigm

As described above, the 1984 report *Physicians for the Twenty-First Century*, issued by the AAMC, included a recommendation that questioned the very basis of the premedical paradigm: "Some institutions may wish to experiment by not recommending any specific course requirements."

In 1965, McMaster University in Hamilton, Ontario, established a new medical school. Now named the Michael G. DeGroote School of Medicine, the new medical school admitted its first class in 1969.[26] McMaster approached medical education in a manner that differed in a number of ways from the approach of other medical schools in Canada or the United States at that time. The medical school adopted a continuous three-year curriculum rather than the standard four-year curriculum. McMaster was a pioneer in adopting a problem-based approach to medical education, an approach that has since been widely adopted by other medical schools. It does not list any specific premedical course requirements for admission.

From its inception, the goal of McMaster was to train "good doctors" for the people of Ontario. In 1972 Hamilton described how the faculty interpreted this charge: "In the elusive 'good doctor,' there are two interwoven sets of qualities: the one, traditional academic qualities, and the other personal qualities of motivation, initiative, and social awareness."[27] Rather than listing any premedical course requirements, McMaster's admissions Web page states, "The intention of the Michael G. DeGroote School of Medicine is to prepare students to become physicians who have the capacity and flexibility to select any area in the broad field of medicine. The applicant is selected with this goal in mind."[28] In its first decade, about one-third of entering medical students had little if any undergraduate instruction in the traditional premedical sciences.[29] Currently about 20 percent of entering students lack the traditional premedical sciences.[30]

McMaster does require clear evidence of academic ability in the students it selects for admission. It measures this academic ability by using the applicant's overall undergraduate GPA without specific regard to courses taken or undergraduate major. In a paper from 1974 describing the "McMaster Philosophy," Neufeld and Barrows described the personal, noncognitive qualities valued by the school and therefore used in selecting students for admission: "demonstrated abilities for independent learning, for imaginative problem-solving, . . . emotional stability, responsibility, motivation for a medical career, and the capacity for self-appraisal."[31] These standards are part of a two-step admissions process developed when the school first opened and still in use today.

As the first step in the admissions process, McMaster obtains an applicant's undergraduate GPA and his or her autobiographical submission to the Ontario Medical School Application Service (a centralized application service similar to the American Medical College Application Service administered by the AAMC). Students are rank-ordered based on a z-scored combination of GPA and autobiographical submission. (Students who have had additional experience as a graduate student receive a slight bonus in the ranking.) The school then invites a predetermined number of these students to campus for an interview based on their initial rank-ordered position. Using the outcomes of the on-campus interview process, a second rank-ordered list of interviewees is created. Students are offered admission based on their position on this second list.

In the overall process of selecting students to whom an offer of admission is made, McMaster gives equal weight to measures of cognitive and noncognitive skills. McMaster has enacted the theoretical model described earlier in figure 5.3; however, they have done so in a way that measures overall academic strengths independent of any specified premedical curricular content. By giving approximately equal weight to cognitive and noncognitive qualities in the selection of applicants for medical school, and by viewing as essentially equal from a cognitive perspective an applicant who has majored in advanced biology with a 3.8 GPA with one who has majored in philosophy with a 3.8 GPA (even though the philosophy student has not taken any courses in chemistry, biology, or physics), McMaster has consciously chosen not to follow the dominant paradigm of premedical education. The obvious question arises: What effect has this choice had on the quality of the students trained at McMaster?

It became apparent early on to researchers and educators at McMaster that the 20–30 percent of students who entered medical school with essentially no science background had a harder time in the first year of so of medical school than did students who entered with an extensive science background. In 1976 Hamilton summarized the early experiences of these students:

> For many, there is essentially no problem. They recognize that they will need to work hard in the basic science areas and organise their work accordingly. Others work well, but suffer in the process and take about a year before they feel fully comfortable. The source of their discomfort is often not a real difficulty, but a sense of insecurity. This derives variously from the difficulty they have in joining in discussions with their science colleagues. Usually this is a matter of familiarity with topic matters and terminology rather than fundamental insights into principles. . . . In general, the difficulty of the non-biological science students seems to diminish by the middle [of the second year].[32]

While acknowledging the difficulties that the non-science students sometimes face, Hamilton also commented on problems encountered with some of the students with a strong science background: "I have personally found most difficulty with students with degrees in physiology or biology who have learnt the stories but not the critical discipline of science and who cannot re-examine their preconceptions. These students are unaware of their own insecurity but create insecurity in others by turning the discussion to matters of detail and 'fact.'"[33] In the context of McMaster's pioneering problem-based curriculum, it appears that too much science was just as likely to cause problems as not enough science.

The issue of the impact of the admissions process with its lack of science prerequisites on the ultimate clinical skills of the students selected for admission was evaluated by Woodward and McAuley.[34] They gathered evaluations from the internship supervisors of 368 recent McMaster graduates, rating the young doctors on eight aspects of competence, then compared the evaluation profile of students who had completed the traditional premedical science curriculum, students who had partially completed that curriculum, and students who had no science courses as an undergraduate. (The internship supervisors were unaware of the premedical background of the interns they were evaluating.) The authors found no difference in the competency ratings among these groups of students.

Of further interest are the results of a question added to the evaluation of the last cohort of students in the study. This question asked the internship supervisor to rate the intern specifically on "knowledge of basic concepts and principles of basic medical science important to patient care." As with the other eight measures of competence, the internship supervisors saw no difference among the student groups in this area of competence. Based on these results and those reported earlier by Hamilton, Woodward and McAuley were able to report: "Taken together, the data we have gathered suggest that medical schools can expand their admissions criteria without feeling that the final product will be inferior because of the lack of traditional preparation for medical school."[35]

In interviews with administrators at McMaster today, the picture described above remains accurate. Many of the approximately 20 percent of students admitted who do not have a strong undergraduate science background have to work harder in the first year to year-and-a-half to catch up to their classmates. However, once they do, they become largely indistinguishable in terms of performance. A few of these students do experience academic difficulty early in their medical school experience.

It will be valuable to focus our attention for a moment on the original methodology with which McMaster measured noncognitive strengths as described by Neufeld and Barrows in 1974. In evaluating an applicant's noncognitive strengths, each applicant's autobiographical submission was reviewed and scored by a three-member team, with one member from the faculty, one from the student body, and one from the community. In subsequently constructing the rank-ordered list for offers of admission, candidates selected for an admissions interview were evaluated in a two-step process: a typical, face-to-face interview with a three-person team representing the same three constituencies, followed by a simulated tutorial in which a group of six applicants was observed, often through a one-way glass, while they discussed a pre-assigned health problem. This second step was intended to measure a candidate's skills in communicating in a group context.

As any advisor to premedical students is well aware, an applicant's written personal statement and responses to written questions submitted as part of the admissions package often undergo multiple drafts, frequently involving input from multiple reviewers. Hanson and colleagues have questioned the validity of such written autobiographical submissions.[36] For the 2005 admissions cycle at McMaster, all applicants submitted written answers to five questions as part of their autobiographical submission. Those candidates selected for an on-campus interview were then asked, while on campus, to submit written answers to eight questions in a time-limited context. Candidates' scores on the questions written off-site were then compared to their scores on the questions written on-site. While the average scores given to the off-site submissions were higher than those for the on-site submissions, the two scores were uncorrelated. The authors concluded that the evidence was "weak" that the written answers submitted for the off-site questions were actually answered independently by the applicants and raised the issue of how this process can be improved.

Eva and colleagues have also questioned the reliability and validity of the typical face-to-face on-campus interview in accurately reflecting an applicant's noncognitive strengths. As discussed in chapter 5, there is considerable research questioning the inter-rater accuracy and test-retest reliability of the interview process and the predictive validity of the score resulting from it. Eva and colleagues posited that the admissions interview, like the traditional clinical oral examination, was limited by the context specific to that one interaction and that by taking multiple "biopsies" instead of one large "chunk," a more reliable and valid measure could be derived. Accordingly, researchers at McMaster developed and extensively tested a multiple mini-interview assessment tool, which they refer to as "an admissions OSCE [objective structured clinical examination]."[37]

As described by Eva and colleagues, the multiple mini-interview (MMI) involves an applicant's going sequentially to seven or more different stations, each set up in a different room. At each station the applicant is given a card explaining the context of the station. Sometimes a trained actor will be part of that context, analogous to the standardized patient of the OSCE. The following are examples of the types of questions and issues posed to applicants:

Station A: Parking Garage. The parking garage at your place of work has assigned parking spots. On leaving your spot, you are observed by the garage attendant as you back into a neighbouring car, a BMW, knocking out its left front headlight and denting the left front fender. The garage attendant gives you the name and office number of the owner of the neighbouring car, telling you that he is calling ahead to the car owner, Tim. The garage attendant tells you that Tim is expecting your visit.

Enter Tim's office. [Tim is an actor]

Station B: Air Travel. Your company needs both you and a co-worker (Sara, a colleague from another branch of the company) to attend a critical business meeting in San Diego. You have just arrived to drive Sara to the airport.

Sara is in the room. [Sara is an actress who explains to you that she has a fear of flying and does not want to go on the trip.][38]

At both stations, the applicant's interaction is observed by a trained evaluator. Other stations might not involve actors; rather, they would involve the evaluator posing a question pertaining to an issue of ethics or one's knowledge of the health care system. Each station lasts no more than eight minutes. The evaluator then rates the applicant, using a 7- or 10-point scale. An aggregate score for each applicant is computed by combining the scores of all stations.

In a research context, Eva and colleagues compared the results of the MMI with those for the traditional interview format. The overall test-retest reliability for the MMI was significantly higher than that for the traditional interview. There was no significant correlation between an applicant's MMI score and his or her score on the traditional interview or his or her undergraduate GPA. (In the years when the MMI was being evaluated in a research context, an applicant's MMI score was not actually used in the admissions decision.)

In follow-up research, Eva and colleagues evaluated the association between a student's MMI score and that student's performance in medical school. Consistent with the research discussed in chapters 4 and 5, the MMI was a strong predictor of a student's score on the OSCE, while a student's undergraduate GPA predicted how well a student would do on multiple choice examinations of medical knowledge.[39] They subsequently followed students through their clinical years, evaluating the association between the MMI and a student's clinical skills.[40] They re-confirmed that the MMI was the best predictor of a student's OSCE score. They also found that the MMI predicted a student's performance on the following sections of the Medical Council of Canada Qualifying Examination (analogous to the USMLE in the U.S.): Population Health; the Considerations of the Legal, Ethical and Organisational Aspects of Medicine; and Clinical Decision Making. The MMI most strongly predicted students' performance in clinical clerkships. While a student's undergraduate GPA predicted his or her performance on a 180–item multiple-choice test used to evaluate a student's scientific and clinical knowledge, the GPA had no power to predict the outcomes associated with the MMI. Based on the outcomes of this research, McMaster now relies heavily on the MMI in evaluating the noncognitive strengths of applicants invited for an interview.

The researchers at McMaster have identified a core principle of the medical school admissions process that reinforces the conclusions drawn from the discussion in chapter 5: "If personal qualities are domains deemed vital to the selection of medical students, then a sufficiently reliable measure of those domains must be applied if an appropriate counterbalance is to be struck with reliably measured cognitive qualities."[41]

For more than four decades, McMaster has followed an approach to premedical education that essentially equates the value of cognitive abilities and noncognitive abilities in the selection of applicants for admission. In the evaluation of cognitive ability, McMaster has focused on overall academic performance, with no additional weight and no specific requirements for courses in chemistry, biology, or physics. They have been able to evaluate noncognitive ability using the MMI instrument they developed.

In an interview with Dr. Harold Reiter, chair of MD admissions at McMaster, I asked for his reaction to the concept of approaching the traditional premedical sciences in an integrated, problem-based curriculum rather than continuing to offer them as individual free-standing subjects. In response, he asked why any predefined curriculum is necessary. If students elect not to take science as an undergraduate, let them do so and then get the needed science as part of medical school. So long as the person is a strong student as reflected by the overall GPA, he or she will be able to catch up in medical school (though also required to work harder than other classmates) and will become fully qualified as a physician.

In choosing not to follow the dominant paradigm of premedical education, McMaster has not sacrificed any increment of quality in the clinical and professional skills of their graduates. Their success in this regard can only call into question the continued appropriateness of the premedical paradigm followed by most other medical schools and undergraduate institutions.

CHAPTER EIGHT

Reassessing the Premedical Paradigm

I began this book by describing the experiences of students I have taught at Stanford over the past 15 years. Early in that teaching experience I recognized a pattern. Students often came to my office to discuss their academic and career plans. As part of these discussions, a number of students would describe how their interest in a career as a physician, an interest they brought with them when they first entered Stanford as a freshman, had now diminished or disappeared altogether. They would often share with me their disappointment at feeling the necessity of giving up those aspirations. These students seemed more often to be female than male; they often were from an underrepresented racial or ethnic minority group (URM). Based on these early impressions, I initiated the research I have described in chapter 1.

From my research I learned that between 2001 and 2005, an average of 363 incoming Stanford freshmen per year indicated on the university's freshman survey an interest in a career as a physician. I also learned that between 2001 and 2008 an average of 294 students per year who had graduated from Stanford University submitted an application to medical school through the American Medical College Application Service operated by the Association of American Medical Colleges (AAMC). It is not at all unexpected that fewer students would apply to medical school than start premedical studies as freshmen. Naturally, some students change their minds over the four years of college. Likewise, it is normal for some students who were not premed as freshmen to decide at some later point to apply to medical school. However, I found that this attrition from premedical studies takes place disproportionately within two groups: URM students and women.

Each year at Stanford, an average of 108 URM students enter freshman year with an interest in medicine. Each year, an average of only 50 URM students apply to medical school—a loss of 58 former premeds from the applicant pool. When we look at non-URM student cohorts, we see a very different outcome. While an average of 255 non-URM students enter Stanford as freshman with an interest in premedical studies, an average of 244 non-URM students apply to medical school each year. For both URM and non-URM cohorts, this decrement occurs disproportionately among women.

Why do women and URM students, all of whom were among the most academically and personally talented high school students in the nation, lose interest in medicine substantially more often than men and non-URM students? Overwhelmingly, the answer is exemplified in this quote, taken from an interview with one of our student-subjects: *"Everyone says it's more like a weeding-out process than anything and I just ended up being one of those people."*

The "it" in this case is the premedical science curriculum, and in particular chemistry courses. Students mentioned chemistry four times more often than any other course as having discouraged their interest in a medical career. Another student responded during her interview: *"I felt that the chemistry courses were designed to weed people out and allows a kind of disconnect between the courses that the people had to take for the premed requirements and the actual type of medicine or career interest they wanted to pursue."*

Contrast this student's experience with the policy advice offered to undergraduate institutions in 1953 by Dr. Aura Severinghaus of Columbia College of Physicians and Surgeons as part of the Report of the Subcommittee on Preprofessional Education of the Survey of Medical Education: *"Effort should be made as early in the student's college career as possible to determine whether, on the basis of personality, character, motivation, and academic performance, he is qualified to go into medicine. If it is decided he is not qualified, then every intelligent device, including aptitude and interest tests, should be used to persuade him to reevaluate his professional objective."*[1]

At Stanford, women and URM students are disproportionately discouraged from persisting in their interest in becoming physicians, with the result that women and URM students are substantially less likely to apply to medical school. The principal factor leading to this loss is the way chemistry, and to a lesser extent the other premedical sciences, are taught. Whether willingly or not, chemistry faculty and chemistry courses carry out the charge given to them in 1953 to persuade these students to reevaluate their professional objective.

Why do we rely on chemistry along with biology and physics to perform this weeding function? This was the question with which I ended chapter 1. To find the answer, it was necessary to go back to the 1870s. In 1873, none of the three medical schools we have been following as exemplars that were then in existence had any requirements for admission other than Michigan's expectation that students complete high school and provide "evidence of a good moral and intellectual character." In that year the University of California had hired Daniel Coit Gilman as its president, and Gilman took charge of the organization of the university's new medical school in San Francisco. Gilman tried unsuccessfully to get the university to adopt preparation in the sciences as a prerequisite for entry into the new medical school. In the face of this resistance, Gilman chose instead to move to the helm of the recently opened Johns Hopkins University in Baltimore. He proposed to the Johns Hopkins trustees the same standard he had proposed in California. This time, the Hopkins trustees supported him, and in 1877 the university's curricular bulletin described what the university considered to be the optimal preparation for the study of medicine: "Physics, Chemistry, and Biology, with Latin, German, French, English form the principal elements of this course."[2] When the Johns Hopkins School of Medicine opened in 1893, all entering students were required to have college-level courses in chemistry, biology, and physics, as well as courses in French and German.

By 1905 Gilman's model of premedical education came to be seen as the new standard of premedical education, and it received the endorsement of the newly created Council on Medical Education (CME). Any medical school that had failed to adopt this standard was graded down in the CME's 1907 report on the quality of medical schools. When Flexner published his report in 1910, the same standard was applied. Failure to enforce this standard of admission was seen as a breach in quality. Of the six exemplar medical schools we have followed in this book, by 1910 all six had adopted the CME standard of requiring chemistry, biology, and physics as prerequisites for admission.

When in the 1920s there were for the first time more applicants to medical school than there were places, science aptitude became the major means of identifying those students most likely to fail the first year of medical school. As a consequence of the rapid movement to a science-based medical school curriculum, as many as one in four entering students at that time failed the first year of medical school. In order to avoid this "wastage" (as it was commonly referred to), the first iteration of what was to become the MCAT was developed and administered. From that point on, the likelihood that a student would encounter academic difficulty in the first year or two of medical school became the principal criterion for selection, and a student's grade point average (GPA) in the premedical sciences combined with his MCAT science scores became the principal means of evaluating this criterion.

By the 1950s, the failure rate in medical school had been reduced dramatically. With the surge in new applicants that followed World War II, there were many more applicants, many of whom were likely to succeed in medical school based on their GPA and MCAT scores. The issue became one of selecting among students, few of whom risked academic failure. For better or for worse, relative performance in the same premedical curriculum as that established in 1893 at Johns Hopkins, measured with essentially the same instruments as those created in the 1920s, was used to select students for admission. The better a student did in the premedical sciences, the better his chance of admission. It was widely assumed that increased performance in the premedical sciences would translate into increased clinical and professional quality among medical graduates. An unfortunate result of this increasing emphasis on grade and test scores was an increasing sense of competition among premedical students—the "premedical syndrome." As described in 1955 by Daniel Funkenstein, at Harvard Medical School the premedical student "becomes more and more anxiety ridden as he contemplates the almost super-human test before him of securing entrance to medical school."[3]

A series of committees and panels of medical educators studied this issue in the years following Funkenstein's description. A general consensus emerged that rather than focusing exclusively on the premedical sciences as undergraduates, medical students should instead bring with them "evidence of a balanced education, as well as demonstrated interest and ability in the natural sciences," as described in 2000 the bulletin of Columbia's medical school. Many medical schools encouraged students to consider non-science majors.

Despite this encouragement, our research has found that, at least at Stanford University and the University of California, Berkeley, incoming freshmen who aspire to become physicians face substantial pressure to enter the established premedical curriculum early in their college career. The first step in that process is to enroll in a series of courses in chemistry. For many students, most of whom are either female or from a URM group or both, that is also an important turning point in their academic and professional career. Their experience in the chemistry classroom conveys to these students the unmistakable message that they are not, as described by Daniel Coit Gilman in the 1870s, "fit to study medicine."

The Origins of the Premedical Paradigm

Why are students at UC Berkeley and Stanford so powerfully affected by early courses in chemistry? If we have known for fifty years or more that chemistry and other premedical science courses are used to sort students into the categories of "fit" and "unfit" to study medicine, why do we still use them in this way in light of their disparate impact on women and URM students?

As the discussion of the history of medical and premedical education included in chapters 2 and 3 suggests, our approach to premedical education today follows a basic model first set in place more than one hundred years ago. That model represented a fundamental change from what had gone before. In 1873, more than thirty years before the CME institutionalized the chemistry-biology-physics model of premedical education we still follow today, the common perception was that, beyond having completed a reasonably high-quality high school education, the principal qualifications for medical school were aspects of one's character, described by the 1873 bulletin of the University of Michigan as including "satisfactory evidence of a good moral and intellectual character." Armed with good moral and intellectual character and an adequate high school education, nearly any student (at least any student who could afford to pay tuition) was eligible to enroll in medical school. Medical science was seen as the collected wisdom of current practitioners. The knowledge base of medical science could be conveyed in a two-year course of clinical instruction.

By 1905, the entire nature of medical science had changed in the United States. A new model of medical education had emerged, involving a minimum four-year curriculum, the first two of which were spent in an intense study of medical science and which relied heavily on laboratory science as a core element of the medical pedagogy. This new model represented not only a fundamentally different structure of medical education but a fundamentally different belief as to what constituted medical knowledge and by what criteria a medical practitioner was to be judged. Over a period of thirty years a revolution had taken place in American medical education.

In 1962 Thomas Kuhn, a professor of the history of science at UC Berkeley, published an important work, *The Structure of Scientific Revolutions,* in which he described the way the perception of "scientific truth" can, from time to time, change fundamentally. Kuhn described this process of change in scientific understanding in the following terms:

> In these and other ways, normal science repeatedly goes astray. And when it does —when, that is, the profession can no longer evade anomalies that subvert the existing tradition of scientific practice—then begin the extraordinary investigations that lead the profession at last to a new set of commitments, a new basis for the practice of science. The extraordinary episodes in which that shift of professional commitments occurs are the ones known in this essay as scientific revolutions. They are the tradition-shattering complements to the tradition-bound activity of normal science.[4]

Between 1873 and 1905, medical science in the United States underwent a revolution—a series of "extraordinary episodes" that resulted in "a new basis for the practice of [medical] science." While Kuhn did not look specifically at the revolution in medical science that took place during this time period, his analysis of the characteristics of previous similar revolutions holds direct relevance for our discussion. Kuhn described certain core characteristics of previous scientific revolutions:

Their achievement was sufficiently unprecedented to attract an enduring group of adherents away from competing modes of scientific activity. Simultaneously, it was sufficiently open-ended to leave all sorts of problems for the redefined group of practitioners to resolve. Achievements that share these two characteristics I shall henceforth refer to as "paradigms," a term that relates closely to "normal science." By choosing it, I mean to suggest that some accepted examples of actual scientific practice—examples which include law, theory, application, and instrumentation together—provide models from which spring particular coherent traditions of scientific research.[5]

In the more than four decades that followed the original publication of Kuhn's theories, there has been a great deal of debate among historians and philosophers of science as to the accuracy and applicability of his theories. Without attempting to resolve this continuing debate, it is nonetheless useful to apply Kuhn's analytic lens to our study of premedical education.

The revolution that took place in premedical education between 1873 and 1905 was no less profound that that which took place during the same time period in medical education and in medical practice. The shift of the standard for premedical education from "satisfactory evidence of a good moral and intellectual character" (as required in 1873 by Michigan) to evidence of the mastery of "the facts of the biological, physical, and chemical sciences [without which] everything that goes under the name of medicine is fraud, sham and superstition" (as argued by Victor Vaughan in 1914) was a revolution equally as profound as was the shift in medical education from a one- or two-year proprietary curriculum to a minimum four-year university-based curriculum.

Kuhn assigns a certain element of chance to the revolutionary process in science. "An apparently arbitrary element, compounded of personal and historical accident, is always a formative ingredient of the beliefs espoused by a given scientific community at a given time."[6] Let us recall the association of Daniel Coit Gilman, M. Carey Thomas, and Mary Garrett surrounding the founding of the Johns Hopkins School of Medicine and the crucial role their association played in establishing both the four-year curriculum at the new medical school and the approach to premedical education that was to become the norm nationally and remains the norm today.

As proposed by Gilman, and with the support of Victor C. Vaughan of Michigan, Charles Eliot of Harvard, and organizations such as the American Academy of Medicine, the American Medical Association, and the Association of American Medical Colleges, a premedical curriculum consisting of prescribed courses in chemistry, biology, physics, and, initially, foreign languages became a model that was to be emulated by nearly all U.S. medical schools. By "attract[ing] an enduring group of adherents away from competing modes of scientific activity" while also leaving open "all sorts of problems for the redefined group of practitioners to resolve" (Kuhn's definitional criteria for a paradigm) this model became the new paradigm of premedical education.

Kuhn's thesis supports the discussion of the previous chapter regarding the dual nature of a paradigm: "On the one hand, it stands for the entire constellation of beliefs, values, techniques, and so on shared by the members of a given community. On the other, it denotes one sort of element in that constellation, the concrete puzzle-solutions which, employed as models or examples, can replace explicit rules as a basis for the solution of the remaining puzzles of normal science."[7] Thus, a paradigm includes two distinct aspects. It is both a statement of a common understanding among scientists of "what the world is like,"[8] and a set of specific models of behavior that create "a new and more rigid definition of the field."[9]

Clearly, the medical educators who established the CME in 1905 had in mind the promulgation of both a new worldview of premedical education and a set of structures and required behaviors defining new standards for premedical education. The publication in 1907 of the CME's analysis of existing medical schools, assigning each of them to one of three categories (acceptable, doubtful, and unacceptable) based to a large degree on whether the school had adopted the CME's standards for premedical education, exemplified both the new worldview and the new standard of practice. When, in 1910, Abraham Flexner in essence replicated the CME's study using the CME's standards for premedical education, he was breaking little new ground, but rather he was disseminating to a substantially wider audience the premedical paradigm promulgated by the CME and its participating organizations.

From this perspective, it is easy to understand why, by the time Vaughan spoke in 1914, the six medical school exemplars followed in previous chapters had adopted a single model of required premedical education—the model defined by the CME as part of the new paradigm. It is also not surprising that this paradigm has persisted largely intact through most of the twentieth century and into the twenty-first. In 2008, more than 90 of medical schools in the United States still adhered to both the worldview that it represents and the standard structure that it brings to the medical school admission process.

Initial Questioning of the Premedical Paradigm

Despite the creation of a new paradigm of premedical education that attracted an "enduring group of adherents," not all observers were fully in support of it and its effects. Recall from chapter 3 that in 1914, the same year Victor Vaughan spoke so stridently in support of the paradigm, Lawrence Lowell, president of Harvard University, argued against expecting college freshmen to focus on completing their premedical requirements early in their college career at the expense of their broader education.

The issue identified by Lowell in 1914 became increasingly problematic in the years following the promulgation of the new paradigm. It was of such concern that in 1925 the AAMC created its own Commission on Medical Education with the charge of reassessing the recent changes that had taken place. Lawrence Lowell was selected as the chairman of the commission. While the commission was generally in support of the new paradigm of medical education, in its 1932 *Final Report*, it spoke critically of the changes that had taken place in premedical education. It concluded that the new premedical requirements "have been rigidly enforced so that at the present time the minimum premedical training is quite uniform in regard to courses."[10] The report speaks firmly in support of the importance of a broad general education in preparation for medical school: "The tendency of medical schools and regulatory bodies to define in detail the range and character of premedical preparation is contrary to the spirit of real education, which should be general and not preprofessional in purpose. A sound general education is of more value to students of medicine than a narrow technical training in the premedical sciences."[11]

Compare these comments with those made in the 1953 report of the Survey of Medical Education: "What kind of education should a preprofessional student have? . . . Some favor a broad liberal education; others, however, give their support to a policy of segregation or semisegregation of preprofessional students and their exposure to a more or less rigid and highly specialized program. . . . [T]he Subcommittee on Preprofessional Education holds that the former affords for greater promise than the latter of developing the prospective doctor into the kind of rounded, balanced, and effective physician whom society needs."[12]

These same cautions were repeated in 1984. In a report titled Physicians for the Twenty-First Century, Stephen Muller, president of Johns Hopkins University and chairman of the AAMC panel that developed the report, cautioned educators that "we perceive a continuing erosion of general education for physicians, an erosion that has not been arrested but [is] instead accelerating. We see continuing pressures to which we must accommodate with vigor and deliberate determination lest critical and irreversible damage be done."[13]

Students at Stanford University and the University of California, Berkeley who enter as freshmen hoping to become physicians know full well what steps they must take to realize their dream. First they must take chemistry—at least two years—and then, at a minimum, a year of biology and a year of physics. Each of these courses must include a laboratory experience. This is what the admissions page of each of our six exemplar medical schools states, this is what the AAMC states, and this is what more than 90 percent of medical schools in the United States expect. Students are often encouraged to consider a non-science major and to value a broad liberal education, but they still must take chemistry, biology, and physics in order to be competitive for medical school. This is the premedical paradigm that defines both a worldview and a set of expected behaviors.

The problem, of course, is that there are many areas in which the paradigm is weak or inadequate when confronted by scientific data. In previous chapters we have identified many of these weaknesses and inadequacies. For example:

- The premedical paradigm holds that, as Flexner stated in 1910, "the normal rhythm of physiologic function must then remain a riddle to students who cannot think and speak in biological, chemical, and physical language."[14] Yet in our review in chapter 4 of nearly a century of data evaluating the association between performance in the premedical sciences and performance as a physician, we find only an indirect relationship. Performance in the premedical sciences, as measured by undergraduate grades or MCAT science scores, is associated with performance in the preclinical sciences taught in medical school but has little if any association with ultimate performance as a physician.

- The premedical paradigm prescribes certain courses and scientific competencies as necessary for the successful study of medicine. However, as T. R. McConnell of UC Berkeley stated in 1957, "In the case of medicine . . . we have the problem of predicting at least two things: first, success in medical school, and second, professional performance."[15] Success in the premedical sciences does not predict professional performance. As discussed in chapters 4 and 5, overall verbal ability and a range of noncognitive strengths largely divorced from the premedical sciences are what best predict ultimate professional performance.

- Finally, as shown in chapter 1, the premedical paradigm affects different social groups differently, with outcomes that are contrary to widely accepted public policy goals. The rigid expectation that students succeed initially in chemistry, and subsequently in biology and physics, leads directly to otherwise qualified students at major universities such as Stanford and UC Berkeley deciding to turn away from medicine as a career. Those students who turn away based on their early experiences in the paradigmatic curriculum are more likely to be female and they are more likely to come from a URM group.

Thus, the premedical paradigm acts as a substantial impediment to increasing the racial and ethnic diversity of the medical profession. As described in chapter 6, a substantial list of programs have focused their efforts on training as physicians students who do not fit the paradigm, often because they did not rise to the expected standard of achievement in the premedical sciences. Given appropriate support and the opportunity, these programs have been shown to train physicians whose clinical and professional competence are largely indistinguishable from that of their colleagues.

Shifting the Paradigm

Kuhn is explicit in seeing paradigms as subject to change, given appropriate circumstances: "Like an accepted judicial decision in the common law, [a scientific paradigm] is an object for further articulation and specification under new or more stringent conditions."[16] New paradigms come into being when common understandings based on the previous order no longer hold up to scrutiny. "Scientific revolutions are inaugurated by a growing sense . . . that an existing paradigm has ceased to function adequately in the exploration of an aspect of nature to which that paradigm itself had previously led the way."[17]

At the time of the Flexner Report, the premedical paradigm helped to provide medical education and medical practice with a firm underpinning of science where none had previously existed. In the early years of its existence, the paradigm was useful in avoiding the "wastage" of large numbers of students entering medical school without adequate preparation in the sciences. However, that paradigm has also contributed to an unfortunate narrowing of the undergraduate educational focus of future physicians. Our own data has shown that the paradigm also creates an unfortunate and unnecessary impediment to many students who otherwise possess the noncognitive strengths of personality, character, and motivation that make them superbly suited to medical practice in the twenty-first century. Kuhn suggested that "paradigm-testing occurs only after persistent failure to solve a noteworthy puzzle has given rise to crisis."[18] I suggest that premedical education, and by extension medical education, is facing just such a crisis today.

U.S. society in the twenty-first century needs physicians with a set of skills and characteristics that are fundamentally different from those identified by Flexner as needed by physicians at the opening of the twentieth century. At that time, physicians needed a firm scientific grounding to their education in order to be able to absorb into their practice the rapidly expanding universe of medical and scientific knowledge. Today's physicians also need to understand medical science, but not as a set of isolated disciplines. Rather, they need to appreciate medical science as an integrated body of knowledge that is most useful when placed in the broader context of addressing problems in human health. The problems the physician of the twenty-first century is most likely to encounter will be those of chronic illness to which even the most advanced scientist will often be unable to offer a cure. Confronting chronic illness in the context of constrained financial resources will necessitate that young physicians acquire a core set of interpersonal skills that they can then couple with their understanding of medical science as an integrated body of knowledge.

Increasingly, medical education is shifting from a discipline-based curriculum to an integrated, problem-based model of learning. The teaching innovations developed by McMaster University and other leading medical schools have become widespread. The premedical preparation today's students will need differs in fundamental ways from the preparation espoused as part of the scientific revolution that was in progress at the opening of the twentieth century.

Physicians in Flexner's time needed laboratory skills in order to conduct their practice. Most of today's physicians have little use for laboratory techniques; rather, they need a thorough understanding the scientific method and the use of statistics in order critically to evaluate research done by others. Physicians in the time of Flexner were predominantly white males. Physicians today are as likely to be female as male and are increasingly needed to represent the growing diversity of our society. Medicine has changed profoundly in the one hundred years since Flexner, and the type of person best suited to become a physician has also changed.

As we saw in chapter 3, the Flexner Report had a profound impact on common perceptions of medical and premedical education even though it broke little new ground. In his report, Flexner replicated a study first done by others affiliated with the CME, those others bringing with them a clearly defined view of the medical world. Flexner adopted that view and laid out his parameters of quality according to them. Physicians and educators adopted both the worldview and the structure of premedical education proposed by Flexner—the premedical paradigm. One hundred years has been enough. It is time to shift the paradigm.

I am not suggesting that we seek a new revolution of premedical education such as took place between 1873 and 1905. Nor am I arguing that we abandon the chemistry-biology-physics sequence of courses that, quite frankly, a good many students are very successful in following and completing. I completed it while in college, and it helped me to build a successful medical career. Rather, I am suggesting that we need to loosen the reins of the premedical paradigm, to permit more flexibility in the way students prepare for and are selected for medical school.

In the introduction to this book, I describe a series of students I have worked with, each of whom held initial aspirations of becoming a physician, and each of whom had those aspirations severely challenged. Some persevered, using experience as a graduate student or as a post-baccalaureate student to demonstrate the personal qualities and academic abilities that made them highly suitable to a career as a physicians—even though the chemistry classroom, and in some instances the chemistry professor, had conveyed to these students the message that they were not "fit to study medicine." As described in the introduction, chemistry has become the "sorting hat" of premedical education. In the case of the students I described, the premedical sorting hat got it wrong.

Still another student gave up altogether on her aspirations for a career in medicine, substituting an aspiration for a career in the law. Chemistry has little to say about a student's suitability for the law, as one of the top law schools in the country perceived when it offered her admission. Did the sorting hat get it right in her case, sending her to a career in the law? Or did it get it wrong, discouraging from a medical career someone who was as capable of becoming a physician, given the appropriate opportunity, as she was of becoming an attorney?

There is extensive evidence that the premedical paradigm tends to sort out many students with that precise quality so necessary for successful medical practice described in 1927 by John Wyckoff as "that quality so difficult to define—character."[19] The medical profession of the twenty-first century needs every one of these students to be doctors as much as the profession of the twentieth century needed young scientists to become doctors. To meet that need, we need to rethink premedical education.

In 2008 Dr. Jules Dienstag, dean for medical education at Harvard Medical School, published an article in the *New England Journal of Medicine* calling for a fundamental restructuring of premedical education. Consistent with what we have learned in this book about the history of the premedical paradigm, Dr. Dienstag argues against those who "view the current premedical science requirements—1 year of biology, 2 years of chemistry (especially organic chemistry), 1 year of physics, and, in some schools, 1 year of mathematics—as a necessary gauntlet that thins out the applicant pool." Dienstag continues, "Unfortunately, current college courses that fulfill admissions requirements are not adequately focused on human biology; the topics covered in many courses in chemistry, physics, mathematics, and even biology are so removed from human biologic principles that they offer little value to the premedical—or advanced human biology—student and steal time and attention from more relevant science preparation."[20]

While not calling for a new paradigm of premedical education, Dienstag is calling for a fundamental reorientation and refocusing of the premedical curriculum to one that provides "greater efficiency and a tighter focus on science that 'matters' to medicine." Recognizing the magnitude of the job involved in stimulating a fundamental shift in the premedical paradigm, Dienstag encourages undergraduate institutions to begin the hard work of making premedical education both more rigorous and more relevant: "Those who teach undergraduates should not shy away from the challenge. Medical schools should stimulate colleges to innovate, and premedical students should demand science courses that prepare them directly and efficiently for the advanced study of biology."[21]

Dienstag's comments hold as much significance for medical educators today as did Charles Eliot's comments in his 1870 Presidential Report at Harvard or Daniel Coit Gilman's comments to the Johns Hopkins trustees in 1878. The time has come to rethink the premedical paradigm and to shift to a model that is more appropriate and more relevant to today's medicine and today's students. In the following chapter I describe such a shift.

CHAPTER NINE

Another Way to Structure Premedical Education

I closed the previous chapter by describing the challenge issued to undergraduate colleges and universities by Jules Dienstag of Harvard. Dienstag indicated that the changes he proposed grew at least partially out of his work with a major national commission convened jointly by the AAMC and the Howard Hughes Medical Institute (HHMI) with the goal of undertaking "a joint, comprehensive assessment of the continuum of premedical and medical science education."[1] He described one of the recommendations that would come from that panel: "Premedical requirements for rigid, 1-to-2-year, discipline-specific science courses should give way to more creative and innovative courses that span and unite disciplines, offering a glimpse of the way biologists and physicians actually navigate real-life problems."

The AAMC/HHMI panel published its report in June 2009, urging medical schools to move to using "'science competency' (learner performance), rather than academic courses, as the basis for assessing the preparation of medical school applicants." The report encourages medical schools to evaluate science competency among premedical students "against a set standard or threshold" rather than as a continuous measure of fitness to study medicine. The report also encourages undergraduate institutions "to develop more interdisciplinary and integrative courses that maintain scientific rigor, while providing a broad and strong liberal arts education."[2]

In an editorial commentary published in *Science* magazine, the panel's co-chairs explicitly acknowledge that there will be multiple approaches to teaching undergraduate science and therefore "multiple routes to gaining a competency."[3] They urge undergraduate educators to explore innovative alternatives to the traditional curriculum and pedagogy. Working with colleagues from Stanford University, the University of California Berkeley, and other universities, I have developed a proposal for a new way to organize the teaching of premedical knowledge that I believe is fully consistent with Dienstag's recommendations and the recommendations of the AAMC/HHMC panel.

Note that I said "premedical knowledge," not "premedical science." While certain content areas within the natural sciences of chemistry, biology, and physics are necessary to gain an understanding of the functioning of the human body, knowledge from these three disciplines alone is not sufficient to ensure such an understanding in the context of medical care. The curriculum I propose goes considerably beyond instruction in these traditional premedical sciences.

The sciences of chemistry, biology, and physics have so changed and enlarged over the hundred years since the Flexner Report as to be barely recognizable to a medical scientist from that day. In 1910, instruction in biology dealt largely with the structure and function of different types of organisms. Beyond microscopic examination of the tissues, the biologist had little means of delving into the inner workings of cells and their constituent parts. Similarly, the chemist was interested principally in the identification of compounds and in the reaction between compounds. With the discovery of atomic structure and the delineation of protons, neutrons, and electrons, chemists began to understand matter in substantially greater depth, yet had little means of applying that new knowledge to the study of human life and human health. Physicists were on the verge of a new understanding of the universe through discoveries in quantum mechanics and concepts of relativity. Each science had its core elements of knowledge; each was thought to be essential to the development of medical knowledge; each had little to do with the others. In figure 9.1A below, I illustrate the relationship of these sciences as it existed at the time of the Flexner Report.

In figure 9.1A, each of the three disciplines stands alone; they are shown with no overlap. A biologist of 1910 used little chemical knowledge directly in the study of biology. Likewise, a physicist used little biology in his study of the nature of matter and space. Each discipline had a subset of knowledge within it, the principles of which every doctor must know. However the disciplines did not overlap—there was no intersecting set. In order to gain those principles of scientific knowledge necessary for the practice of medicine, principles that were embedded somewhere in the ovals representing the state of scientific knowledge at the time, each student was required to take a one-year course in each discipline. (The course in chemistry became a two-year course a few years later.)

Now let us fast-forward to the state of scientific knowledge in 2010, one hundred years after the Flexner Report. The associations among chemistry, biology, and physics are illustrated schematically in part B of figure 9.1. We notice some striking differences between the representations of premedical science in the two figures. Each of the disciplines is substantially larger in 2010 than in 1910, representing the tremendous expansion in scientific knowledge that has ensued. Perhaps more im-

A

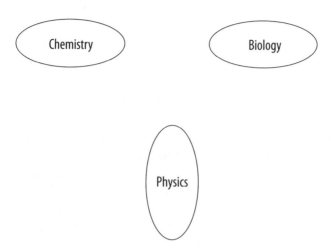

B

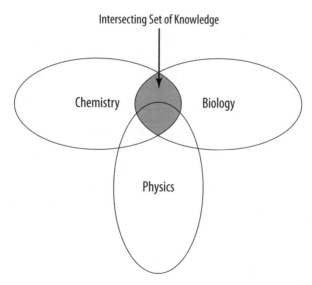

Figure 9.1. The disciplines of premedical science in (A) 1910 and (B) 2010

portantly, as each of the disciplines has expanded, each has grown closer to the other such that they all now overlap. There is subset of knowledge (referred to in the figure as the "intersecting set") that is common either to all three disciplines or to at least two of them. All elements of knowledge in this subset are simultaneously part of more than one discipline.

For example, let us consider the structure of the DNA molecule. DNA is made up of a double helix—two connected rows of molecules wound around each other. DNA is the core element of life, constituting both the means of reproducing life and the means of regulating life. It is made up of a repetitive series of the molecules adenine, cytosine, guanine, and thymine, known as nucleotides. Without going further into the detail of the molecular structure and function of DNA, I will pose this question: If we are studying DNA, are we studying chemistry or are we studying biology? In 1910 chemistry and biology were dichotomous; in 2010 they are, to a substantial extent, continuous. The study of DNA is simultaneously the study of chemistry and the study of biology—it is part of biochemistry. It is part of the intersecting set of the two disciplines.

Let us also consider the flow dynamics of a particular fluid—human blood—in a particular set of tubular structures—human blood vessels. As I learned as part of college physics, the dynamics of the flow of a fluid through a tubular structure will depend on several factors, including the viscosity of the fluid, the diameter (or was it the radius?) of the tube, and the temperature of the surrounding environment. If we study the effects of a narrowing of the diameter of an arteriole (small artery) on the resistance encountered by the blood flowing through the arteriole and the resulting pressure exerted on the wall of the tube, are we studying physics or are we studying biology? We are studying the intersection of the two sciences, and when we add changes in fluid viscosity due to an abnormally high level of glucose in the blood, we are studying chemistry, biology, and physics simultaneously.

Shortly after 1910, when it was decided that chemistry needed to be separated into its constituent parts of inorganic chemistry and organic chemistry, it took a minimum of four years of study to learn the requisite knowledge contained within the three disciplines of premedical science: one year of physics, one year of biology, and two years of chemistry. While that requisite knowledge was certainly learned, so too was a great deal of material that had little to do with medicine. In 1965–66, I took a year-long course in organic chemistry that was required as part of my biology major in college. I can remember clearly one of my most fascinating experiences in that course. By meticulously following the instructions in the laboratory manual, I was able to get two liquids into a beaker, one on top of the other, with a distinct interface between them. If I *ever so carefully* reached into that interface with a pair of tweezers, grabbed it, and slowly pulled the tweezers out of the beaker, a consistent white strand followed the tweezers. I could keep pulling and pulling, and the strand would get progressively longer until all of both liquids in the beaker had been converted into a single, very long, white strand. *I had synthesized nylon!* It was fascinating. Nylon is a polymer; DNA is a polymer. I learned the basic principles of polymerization in a few minutes of lecture and a few pages of the text. The several additional hours it took for me to make my strand of nylon were thoroughly enjoyable (at least to me—not all of my classmates had the same success). Synthesizing nylon may have been fascinating, but it had little if anything to do with medicine. I can say this definitively after more than thirty years of medical practice. The knowledge of polymer chemistry, beyond a basic understanding of the concept, is not part of the intersection of scientific sets that comprises necessary premedical knowledge.

What if, rather than teaching premedical students all about polymer chemistry as well as about all other aspects of chemistry, biology, and physics, we instead teach them only about what is in the intersection of the three disciplines, as represented in figure 9.1B? Would we be diminishing their scientific knowledge such that their chance of successfully completing the first year or two of medical school was correspondingly diminished? Quite the contrary, the data described in the earlier chapters of this book suggest that, armed with the knowledge contained within the intersecting set, they would do quite well in medical school, assuming they had also demonstrated a general academic ability and the aspects of personality, character, and motivation required for success in medicine.

Structure and Content of the Proposed Curriculum

The time has come to develop such a course on a pilot basis and to offer it as an experimental alternative to the traditional curriculum that continues to follow the premedical paradigm described by Flexner. What should we call such a course? It is neither chemistry, nor is it biology, nor is it physics. It is a part of each but synonymous with none. Accordingly, I suggest we name the intersecting set of these three disciplines the "human life sciences." Within this concept I include

- *Human Biology:* those aspects of biology that are integral to understanding the structure and function of the human organism
- *Chemistry:* those principles of inorganic and organic chemistry necessary to gain a full understanding of human biology
- *Physics:* those principles of physics necessary to gain a full understanding of human biology

The traditional curriculum for premedical students and for students considering a career in the biomedical sciences includes at least two years of chemistry, one year of biology, and one year of physics, each taught in a separate department. The course I propose would be offered as an alternative to this traditional curriculum. The purpose of the new course is to provide students with a firm grounding in the human life sciences in a single integrated course that uses a curricular and pedagogical structure more appropriate for those students who have traditionally encountered personal discouragement or academic difficulty in the traditional science curriculum. By developing an alternative learning environment based on recent research from social psychology and educational psychology, a goal of this proposal is to increase the diversity of students who select careers in either medicine or the biomedical sciences.

We should be clear on one important aspect of this proposal, however. I began this book with a discussion of the factors that impeded the expansion of the racial and ethnic diversity of entering medical students. It is true that I expect the new course structure to be attractive to many URM students and that, given adequate social and academic support, these and other students who come from disadvantaged educational backgrounds and who take the new course will likely have more success in their premedical studies and will be more likely to persist in those studies and apply to medical school. I also expect the same to be true for many women students who, as our research has shown, interpret unsatisfactory early experiences in the chemistry classroom as a message to find a different career path. However, the new course is not focused solely on the needs of URM students or on the needs of women. It is intended to meet the needs of a wide range of students who enter college with hopes of becoming physicians but who don't fit the mold created by the premedical paradigm.

Let us reconsider the goals and the outcomes of two programs described in chapter 7: the Humanities and Medicine Program (HMP) at the Mt. Sinai School of Medicine, and the admissions polices and procedures followed by McMaster School of Medicine. Neither is intended as a program to increase racial or ethnic diversity among medical students. Neither is intended to be more suitable or attractive to one gender over the other. Rather, both are intended to attract to the study of medicine students with certain noncognitive strengths and characteristics that are often lacking among medical students. As described earlier, HMP has the goal of providing "maximum flexibility in the undergraduate years for students to explore their interests in humanities and social sciences."[4] McMaster seeks as medical students those applicants who bring with them "two interwoven sets of qualities: the one, traditional academic qualities, and the other personal qualities of motivation, initiative, and social awareness."[5]

Figure 5.3 summarized the research findings reviewed in that chapter. In the twenty-first century the optimal physician will bring with him or her a balance of scientific aptitude and personality strengths. Historically, the premedical paradigm has identified those most "fit to study medicine" as students with superior academic ability, with substantially less emphasis placed on their noncognitive aspects. The new curriculum I envision is targeted to those students who fall within the shaded area of figure 5.3 labeled as "Most Highly Qualified," but who do not fit within the concept of "Most Highly Qualified" as generated by the traditional paradigm, illustrated in figure 5.2.

The new curriculum is targeted for all students with both the academic ability and the strength of personality necessary to succeed as physicians, but it will seek out especially those students with these requisite characteristics who otherwise might find themselves "weeded out" by the traditional premedical paradigm. Many of these students will be from URM groups; many will not. Many will be women; many will not. Most will be most comfortable in a learning environment such as that pioneered by McMaster and widely applied in U.S. medical schools today in which new knowledge is placed in the context of a problem of human health and well being rather than being listed on the blackboard.

In order to meet the educational needs of this group of students, I envision that the course will have the following characteristics:

1. The course will be taught by a team of faculty, staff, and graduate students representing the three principal human life sciences disciplines: biology, chemistry, and physics. This team will work collaboratively to design and present the curriculum in a way that conveys accurate scientific knowledge but does so by weaving the three disciplines together. The team will jointly design the means by which student progress will be assessed and by which students who encounter difficulty will be offered additional support.

2. The course will present information from the human life sciences in an integrated fashion, focusing on those scientific principles necessary to understand a given contextual focus. It will not be simply a compendium of traditional premedical courses in chemistry, biology, and physics. Rather, as illustrated in figure 9.1B above, it will identify and teach the knowledge content of the intersection of the knowledge sets that comprises human life sciences as I have defined them.

3. The course will adopt a context-based approach to teaching, analogous to the problem-based learning that has become a common part of the curriculum at many medical schools. For many students, including many women and URM students, problem-based curricula and other similar pedagogies have been shown to more conducive to science learning than the traditional didactic curriculum that relies more heavily on lectures and readings without a contextual framework.[6] For exam-

ple, the pedagogy of the course might be based on the structure of the human organism, addressing in sequence:

a. The cell nucleus, including nucleic acids and the chemical basis of biological information

b. Cell structure and function

c. Organs and organ systems

d. Physiologic and homeostatic systems

e. The human organism and its association with its environment

4. The course will present information from the human life sciences in an integrated fashion, focusing on those scientific principles necessary to understand a given contextual focus. By having an integrated team of instructors, each topic encountered at the various levels of analysis can be addressed either simultaneously or sequentially by instructors with different backgrounds and training.

For example, consider how the topic of the cell membrane might be taught. The cell membrane is typically composed of a combination of protein and lipid molecules. It has a dual function: to hold the contents of the cell in place, and to let selected chemical compounds move in and out of the cell. Having said that, it would be appropriate to diverge for a bit to understand more about the chemistry of lipids and proteins: how are they constructed, how are they similar, how are they different? For this we need to know fundamental principles of chemical bonds between and among molecules. However, we also need to understand the dual functions of the cell membrane of maintaining structure and selectively permitting diffusion across its boundaries. Why is diffusion across cell membranes important to cell functioning? What type of molecules might be involved in this diffusion? How does electrical charge among ions affect this diffusion?

5. The course will rely extensively on electronic teaching aids integrated with didactic and group-based learning. An example of such an electronic teaching resource that might be incorporated into the curriculum is ChemSense®, described as, "an NSF-funded project to study students' understanding of chemistry and develop software and curriculum to help students investigate chemical systems and express their ideas in animated chemical notation."[7] Many of the most exciting advances in college-level instruction involve electronic resources of this type. It is my hope that additional such resources will be developed as part of this curriculum.

I hope it is evident (as I'm confident it is for anyone who has taken a traditional course in organic chemistry) that this approach to teaching and to learning differs fundamentally from the pedagogical approach common to the traditional chemistry, biology, and physics classrooms. I hope it is also evident that an approach such as I have described will be attractive to a diverse groups of students—intellectually diverse as well as diverse in terms of gender and ethnicity—and will help many of these students succeed in their premedical studies who might otherwise have turned away from a medical career.

To complete the premedical sciences that make up the traditional paradigm requires four years of study: two years studying chemistry, one year studying biology, and one year studying physics. These year-long course can be taken sequentially, or, for some brave souls, simultaneously. I expect that the integrated, context-based curriculum outlined above would take two years to complete. Shortening from four years to two the time required to complete the premedical curriculum will realize at least two additional benefits: (1) allowing the students to delay the start of the premedical curriculum until the sophomore or junior year, and (2) enabling students to take additional courses in the social sciences and humanities.

Further Benefits of the Integrated, Context-Based Curriculum

From the research presented in chapter 4, we learned that among the various MCAT sub-tests, the Verbal Ability score is the strongest predictor of a physician's clinical skills as measured by the USMLE-III. Many students, especially students from disadvantaged educational backgrounds, enter college with weak verbal skills relative to their classmates. Many of these are the very students who, when immediately placed in a highly competitive chemistry classroom, encounter difficulty. By delaying the start of the alternative curriculum until the sophomore year (or later), all students, but especially disadvantaged students, will have the opportunity both to strengthen their verbal skills in preparation for medical school and to adapt to the academic and intellectual climate of college.

Recall the comments of Dr. Ezekiel Emanuel cited in chapter 1: "Why are calculus, organic chemistry, and physics still premed requirements? Mainly to 'weed out' students. Surely, it would be better to require challenging courses on topics germane to medical practice, research, or administration to assess the quality of prospective medical students, rather than irrelevant material."[8]

For fifteen years I taught a series of courses to undergraduates at Stanford University, a majority of whom were premedical students. One course explored American health policy; a second course examined the roots of health disparities that lie in factors such as social class, race, and ethnicity. I have heard repeatedly from students who have taken these courses and have then gone to medical school that what they learned in them was directly relevant to their medical education and their medical practice. In addition, I have seen firsthand how courses in biomedical ethics offered by other instructors at Stanford have been equally relevant and useful to students entering medicine. Each student taking the proposed premedical curriculum would be encouraged (perhaps required) also to take courses such as these as part of their preparation for medical school. I heartily concur with Emanuel that courses such as these would be at least as "germane to medical practice, research, or administration" as much of the content of traditional science courses.

As yet I have said little regarding the role of laboratory instruction as part of the proposed curriculum. Repeatedly, throughout the discussion of the history of premedical education summarized in previous chapters, the principal justifications for requiring students to include extensive laboratory experience as part of the premedical curriculum were twofold: to acquire technical laboratory skills necessary for the practice of medicine, and to understand and appreciate the scientific method. I entered medical practice in 1974. For the first several years of my practice as a primary care physician I was capable of performing a few basic blood and urine tests in my office and of staining and examining under the microscope a few types of specimens. A few years into my practice the licensure regulations changed, and I would have had to get a new type of license to perform and charge for these tests. Accordingly, I stopped doing them, coming instead to rely on a hospital lab or private lab locally. I have not carried out a laboratory procedure in its entirety for more than 25 years. My understanding is that few of my medical colleagues, other than pathologists or certain sub-specialists, carry out laboratory procedures as a direct part of their practice. Similarly, I have queried a substantial number of former premedical students who are now medical students. Other than gross anatomy laboratory, where they learn dissection, none has indicated that direct instruction or experience in laboratory techniques or procedures was part of their medical education. It is my sense that, for most physicians, developing advanced laboratory skills and techniques is no longer a relevant part of medical education or medical practice.

Rather, the value of laboratory experience is in learning to appreciate the strengths and the limitations of the scientific method. In defending the role of organic chemistry in the premedical paradigm, Kramer argued that "the critical thinking and problem-solving skills of organic chemistry formed the foundation of my medical training." Higgins and Reed suggest that organic chemistry and physics "contribute a great deal to providing the framework for understanding basic principles of medicine." In defending the inclusion of these sciences, these authors seem to be defending their role in teaching the scientific method more so than their factual or technical content.[9]

I fully concur that we need to teach an understanding and appreciation of the scientific method to all premedical students. However, synthesizing strands of nylon in the organic chemistry lab or, as was my assignment in physics lab, calculating the period of a pendulum, does not accomplish this task. Rather than teaching laboratory technique, the laboratory component of the curriculum I propose is focused on teaching the methodology of science, both its strengths and its weaknesses.

In teaching the scientific method, it will be crucial for students to learn the process of going from an unanswered research question to being able to describe and defend the answer to that question through the analysis of scientific data. It will be important for students to learn how the process differs for questions of social science and questions of genetics or molecular biology. Knowing how to collect data, which data to collect, and what analytic methods to apply to the data are all things that can be learned in both a seminar context and a laboratory context. A fundamental understanding of principles of statistics will be part of this learning process.

Students' knowledge of the scientific method should also be supplemented by an appreciation of its potential weaknesses. What is the role of uncertainty in analyzing data and reporting results? How does one measure the mathematical effects of uncertainty, and how does one measure its psychological effects? These are areas in which instruction in the history and philosophy of science can play crucial roles. Finally, no instruction in research methodology can be complete without a discussion of the ethics of research. In evaluating the results of a project, does it matter how the research was funded? To whom does a scientist owe his or her duty?

As part of the new premedical curriculum, I suggest we replace the previously required four years of experience in a science laboratory with one or two years of study of the scientific method. This instruction will include actual time in a laboratory conducting experiments, and it will include time in a seminar discussing and debating some of the issues described above. I believe that after such instruction a student will be substantially better prepared for the study and practice of medicine than he or she would have been after four years spent doing sequential experiments described in the laboratory manual and overseen by the lab TA.

A question I have not addressed, yet one that is quite germane to our discussion is whether successful completion of the proposed new curriculum will prepare a student equally well to go on to medical school or to go on to graduate school in a biomedical science. I suggest that it would. It is my hope and expectation that a substantial number of students who complete the proposed curriculum will see the importance and the excitement of contributing directly to the expansion of biomedical science in ways that extend our ability to treat illness and injury. I believe that students completing this curriculum who select a research career will be fully capable of going on to take more focused and advanced courses in biochemistry or other biomedical sciences and will be fully capable, with appropriate instruction and mentoring, of initiating a program of laboratory-based scientific research.

Evaluating the Outcomes of the Proposed Curriculum

The premedical curriculum proposed by the CME in 1905 and supported by Flexner in 1910 was, by 1914, adopted as the national standard by which medical schools would be evaluated. It was adopted on the faith that it would provide the optimal preparation for medical school but with essentially no scientific evidence that it actually did so. I suggest that we not repeat this methodological error.

What I have proposed is essentially a research hypothesis:

> H1: *A restructured premedical curriculum will bring a more diverse pool of students into medical school without a decrement in the clinical or professional quality of physicians trained in this manner.*

As with any research hypothesis, this one must be evaluated by well-designed research. Once completed, I believe the research will support the hypothesis. On the other hand, it may not. Thus, in parallel to the revised curriculum itself, I propose an ongoing program of research to evaluate the new curriculum.

As part of this research, I expect several early outcomes:

a. The racial and ethnic diversity of self-declared premedical students electing the new curriculum will be greater than the comparable diversity of students electing the traditional curriculum.

b. Women premedical students will elect the new curriculum more often than the traditional curriculum.

c. Students electing the new curriculum will have a greater range of noncognitive strengths than those electing the traditional curriculum.

A second level of analysis will come after students have completed the curriculum, leading to the testing of the following additional hypothesis:

d. Those students shown in previous research to be more likely to lose interest in continuing in premedical studies (i.e., women, URM students, and students from disadvantaged educational backgrounds) will be more likely to maintain their interest in a medical career and to apply to medical school when compared to comparable students who elect the traditional premedical curriculum.

A third level of analysis will come after graduates of the curriculum have entered and completed at least the first two years of medical school. With the realization that there may be changes soon in the way grades are assigned in medical school and licensure examinations are administered, the next hypothesis may need to be adjusted in light of these changes.

e. Students who complete the new curriculum and enter medical school will perform at least as well as students who took the traditional premedical curriculum, using medical school grades and the results of USMLE-I as measures of performance.

The final comparisons between students taking the new curriculum and those taking the traditional curriculum can only come several years in the future, after both groups of students have completed medical school and entered into residency training and medical practice.

f. Students who complete the new curriculum and complete medical school will demonstrate a level of clinical and professional quality that is at least as high as students from the traditional curriculum, using USMLE-II, USMLE-III, standardized patient performance, and residency evaluations as measures of quality.

g. Students who complete the new curriculum and who enter medical practice will be more likely to elect practice in a primary care specialty than those completing the traditional curriculum.

Of course it will take at least a decade to begin to test these final hypotheses. However, given that the traditional premedical paradigm has been in place for more than one hundred years and still has not been fully supported with scientific evidence, a decade does not seem an overly long time to decide whether a shift in that paradigm such as I propose will attain the goals and outcomes set for it. However, as with many clinical trials, it will be important to set important mid-point evaluations that will enable us to gauge the progress being made toward the goal. If it turns out that, after only a few years, there is no support for hypotheses (a) through (d), it would seem to make little sense to continue the experiment. Thus, I propose to set in place a program of rigorous analysis of the new curriculum from the outset.

The first cohorts of premedical students who take the proposed curriculum as an alternative to the traditional premedical curriculum will face a potential disadvantage in gaining admission to medical school because they will not have taken the specific science courses required for admission by more than 90 percent of U.S. medical schools. In addition, because they have studied only a subset of physics and chemistry, they may not be fully prepared to take the Physical Sciences portion of the MCAT. Accordingly, before initially offering the curriculum on a pilot basis, it will be important to be in contact with the admissions offices of a range of medical schools and with the Association of American Medical Colleges to seek their support for this pilot project and their collaboration in completing the outcomes research that is a crucial part of it.

Since what I propose is a research project, it is incumbent on any participating institution to make any student who elects the new curriculum fully aware that, while there may be substantial benefits to participating in the new curriculum, there may also be risks. Accordingly, the proposal must be thoroughly reviewed by the university's Human Subjects Protection panel and must use written informed consent procedures with every student who elects to enroll. Only in this way will it be possible to fulfill our ethical obligation as researchers to, above all else, protect the well-being of our research subjects—in this case, our students.

Closing Thoughts

In the years following the publication of the Flexner Report in 1910, Abraham Flexner was widely perceived has having set in motion a series of revolutionary changes in both medical education and premedical education. As we have learned from our review of the years preceding and following the issuance of his report, Flexner actually added relatively little in the way of new knowledge or new perspectives to a process of scientific revolution that was already well on its way to completion.

Given the importance of the historical role commonly assigned to the Flexner Report, its centennial year of 2010 will undoubtedly see a spate of commentary and analysis. I hope the review I have presented here will contribute both to this discussion and to the evolutionary changes in premedical education that I believe are already well underway. The premedical paradigm supported by Flexner served us well for much of the twentieth century. I hope and expect that the new, evolving model of premedical education will serve us well in the twenty-first.

Preface

1. T. S. Kuhn, *The Structure of Scientific Revolutions,* 2nd ed. (Chicago: University of Chicago Press, 1970), 175, 5, 19.

Introduction

1. G. H. Breiger, "The Plight of Premedical Education: Myths and Misperceptions—Part I: The Premedical Syndrome," *Academic Medicine* 74 (1999): 901–4.

2. S. Lewis, *Arrowsmith* (New York: Penguin Group, 1998), 7.

3. A. Flexner, *Medical Education in the United States and Canada* (New York: Carnegie Foundation for the Advancement of Teaching, 1910), 23–24.

4. D. H. Funkenstein, "Some Myths about Medical School Admissions," *Journal of Medical Education* 30 (1955): 81.

5. A. E. Severinghaus, H. J. Carmen, and W. E. Cadbury, *Preparation for Medical Education in the Liberal Arts Colleges: The Report of the Subcommittee on Preprofessional Education of the Survey of Medical Education* (New York: McGraw-Hill, 1953).

6. Ibid., 99.

Chapter 1 · Who Drops Out of Premed, and Why?

1. J. J. Cohen, "Finishing the Bridge to Diversity," 1996 AAMC presidential address, p. 1, available at www.aamc.org/diversity/reading.htm.

2. Association of American Medical Colleges, "Diversity in the Physician Workforce: Facts & Figures 2006," p. 9, available at www.aamc.org/diversity.

3. B. D. Smedley, A. Y. Stith, L. Colburn, and C. H. Evans, eds., *The Right Thing to Do, the Smart Thing to Do: Enhancing Diversity in the Health Professions* (Washington, DC: National Academies Press, 2001), 2.

4. Committee on Institutional and Policy-Level Strategies for Increasing the Diversity of the U.S. Healthcare Workforce, Institute of Medicine, *In the Nation's Compelling Interest: Ensuring Diversity in the Health Care Workforce* (Washington, DC: National Academies Press, 2004), 5.

5. Association of American Medical Colleges, "Diversity in the Physician Workforce."

6. University of California, Office of the Vice President for Health Affairs, "Medical Education and the University of California: Final Report of the Health Sciences Committee, 2004."

7. T. Bates and S. Chapman, "Diversity in California's Health Professions: Physicians," UCSF Center for the Health Professions, 2008, available at http://futurehealth.ucsf.edu.

8. K. Grumbach, K. Odom, G. Moreno, E. Chen, C. Vercammen-Grandjean, and E. Mertz, "Physician Diversity in California: New Findings from the California Medical Board Survey," Center for California Health Workforce Studies, University of California, San Francisco, 2008, iv, available at www.futurehealth.ucsf.edu.

9. Ibid., vi.

10. University of California, Office of Health Affairs, Medical Student Diversity Task Force, "Special Report on Medical Student Diversity, 2000," available at www.ucop.edu/healthaffairs/reports/diversity/welcome.html.

11. Data on medical school applicants who had attended Stanford University were provided by the Association of American Medical Colleges.

12. A. A. Summers and B. L. Wolfe, "Estimating Household Income from Location," *Journal of the American Statistical Association* 73 (1978): 288–92.

13. K. Lovecchio and L. Dundes, "Premed Survival: Understanding the Culling Process in Premedical Undergraduate Education," *Academic Medicine* 77 (2002): 719–24.

14. E. J. Emanuel, "Changing Premed Requirements and the Medical Curriculum," *JAMA* 296 (2006): 1128–31; quotation on 1129.

15. Princeton Review, "Premed Requirements," available at www.princetonreview.com/medical/research/articles/criteria/prereqs.asp.

16. Wikipedia, "Premedical," available at http://en.wikipedia.org/wiki/Premedical.

17. Columbia University College of Physicians and Surgeons, "Entrance Requirements," available at www.cumc.columbia.edu/dept/ps/admissions/apply.html.

18. Harvard University Medical School, "Requirements for Admission," available at http://hms.harvard.edu/admissions.

19. Johns Hopkins School of Medicine, "Admissions Requirements," available at www.hopkinsmedicine.org/admissions/apps.html.

20. University of California, San Francisco School of Medicine, "Course Requirements," available at www.medschool.ucsf.edu/admissions/apply/gettingstarted.

21. University of Michigan School of Medicine, "Subject Requirements," available at www.med.umich.edu/medschool/admissions/process/requirements.htm.

22. Stanford University School of Medicine, "Academic Requirements," available at http://med.stanford.edu/md/admissions/preparation.html.

23. Association of American Medical Colleges, "Medical School Admission Requirements, 2008–2009," 11.

24. J. M. Stalnaker and J. Eindhoven, eds., *Admission Requirements of American Medical Colleges* (Chicago: Association of American Medical Colleges, 1951).

25. S. Lewis, *Arrowsmith* (New York: Penguin Group, 1998), 7.

26. D. B. Kramer, T. S. Higgins, V. U. Collier et al., Comments on "Changing Premedical Requirements," *JAMA* 297 (2007): 37–38.

27. A. Flexner, *Medical Education in the United States and Canada* (New York: Carnegie Foundation for the Advancement of Teaching, 1910), 24.

Chapter 2 · The Historical Origins of Premedical Education in the United States, 1873–1905

1. I have reviewed published medical bulletins and additional materials kept in the archives of the Columbia University Medical Center; the Center for the History of Medicine at the Countway Library of Harvard Medical School; the Bentley Historical Library of the University of Michigan; the Alan Mason Chesney Medical Archives of Johns Hopkins University; the Special Collections and Archives of Stanford University; and the Archives & Special Collections of the Medical Library of the University of California, San Francisco.

2. G. H. Breiger, "'Fit to Study Medicine': Notes for a History of Pre-Medical Education in America," *Bulletin of the History of Medicine*, 57 (1983): 6.

3. University of California, San Francisco. A History of the UCSF School of Medicine, available at http://history.library.ucsf.edu.

4. G. H. Breiger, "The California Origins of the Johns Hopkins Medical School," *Bulletin of the History of Medicine* 51 (1977): 349.

5. R. H. Fishbein, "Origins of Modern Premedical Education," *Academic Medicine* 76 (2001): 426.

6. Ibid.

7. P. Starr, *The Social Transformation of American Medicine* (New York: Basic Books, 1982), 113–14.

8. A. Flexner, *Medical Education in Europe*, The Carnegie Foundation for the Advancement of Teaching, Bulletin Number Six, 1912.

9. K. M. Ludmerer, *Learning to Heal: The Development of American Medical Education* (Baltimore: Johns Hopkins University Press, 1996), 48.

10. Ibid.

11. Ibid., 50.

12. Johns Hopkins University Curricular Bulletin, 1877, as quoted by R. H. Fishbein, "Maryland Medical History," *Maryland Medical Journal* 48 (1999): 229.

13. D. C. Gilman, "On the Studies Which Should Precede a Course of Study in Medicine, Hygiene, Etc.," in A. M. Chesney, "Two Documents Relating to Medical Education at Johns Hopkins University," *Bulletin of the Institute of the History of Medicine* IV(6) (1936): 482.

14. D. F. Smiley, "History of the Association of American Medical Colleges, 1876–1956," *Journal of Medical Education* 32 (1957): 512.

15. Ibid., 514.

16. S. J. Peitzman, "Forgotten Reformers: The American Academy of Medicine," *Bulletin of the History of Medicine* 58 (1984): 517–18.

17. American Academy of Medicine, Constitution, *Bulletin of the American Academy of Medicine* I(14) (1893): 284–85.

18. D. S. Jordan, "The General Education of the Physician," *Bulletin of the American Academy of Medicine* I(6) (1891): 14.

19. Ibid., 18.

20. P. S. Conner, "Essentials and Non-essentials in Medical Education," *Bulletin of the American Academy of Medicine* I (10) (1892): 131.

21. H. B. Allyn, "The Value of Academic Training Preparatory to the Study of Medicine," *Bulletin of the American Academy of Medicine* I(11) (1892): 182–84.

22. H. F. Warner, "Discussion of 'The Value of Academic Training Preparatory to the Study of Medicine' by HB Allyn," *Bulletin of the American Academy of Medicine* I(11) (1892): 185.

23. V. C. Vaughan, "Does a Classical Course Enable a Student to Shorten the Period of Professional Study?" *Bulletin of the American Academy of Medicine* I(13) (1893): 225–26.

24. V. C. Vaughan, "The Kind and Amount of Laboratory Work Which Should Be Required in Our Medical Schools," *Journal of the American Medical Association* XIX (1892): 665–67.

25. Gilman, "Studies Which Should Precede a Course of Study in Medicine," 486.

26. Ibid., 488.

27. H. L. Horowitz, *The Power and Passion of M. Carey Thomas* (New York: Alfred A. Knopf, 1994).

28. Ibid.

29. A. M. Chesney, An Account of the Negotiations with Miss Mary E. Garrett Concerning the Terms of Her Gift for the Medical School, November 12, 1942, Alan Mason Chesney Archives, The Johns Hopkins Medical Institutions.

30. M. E. Garrett, Letter to Johns Hopkins University trustees of December 24, 1892, as quoted in D. C. Gilman, Remarks addressed to the Board of Trustees of the Johns Hopkins University and read to them at their meeting, January 3, 1893. Alan Mason Chesney Archives, The Johns Hopkins Medical Institutions.

31. Gilman, Remarks.

32. M. E. Garrett, The Mary Elizabeth Garrett Fund—Terms of the Gift as Accepted by the Trustees, February 21, 1893, *Bulletin of the Johns Hopkins Medical School,* 1894, 17–21, Alan Mason Chesney Archives, The Johns Hopkins Medical Institutions.

33. Ibid., 18.

34. D. C. Gilman, Address given on Commemoration Day, Johns Hopkins University, February 22, 1893. Alan Mason Chesney Archives, The Johns Hopkins Medical Institutions.

35. Association of American Medical Colleges, Transactions—Fifth Annual Session, *Bulletin of the American Academy of Medicine* I(22) (1894): 531–39.

36. Association of American Medical Colleges, Regarding the requirements for admission to be maintained by colleges belonging to the Association, *Journal of the American Medical Association* 37 (1901): 757–62.

37. M. A. Fishbein, *A History of the American Medical Association 1847 to 1947* (Philadelphia: W. B. Saunders Company, 1947), 891.

38. Ibid.

39. A. D. Bevan, Report of the Committee on Medical Education, *Journal of the American Medical Association* 40 (1903): 1372–73.

40. A. D. Bevan, Report of the Committee on Medical Education, *Journal of the American Medical Association* 42 (1904): 1576.

41. Ibid.

42. V. C. Vaughan, "Some Remarks on the Present Status of Medical Education in the United States," *Journal of the American Medical Association* 40 (1903): 1120.

43. G. H. Simmons, "Medical Education and Preliminary Requirements," *Journal of the American Medical Association* 42 (1904): 1207–209.

44. L. S. McMurtry, "Introductory Remarks, First Annual Conference, Council on Medical Education," *Journal of the American Medical Association* 44 (1905): 1470.

45. A. D. Bevan, "The History of the Council and the Scope of Its Work," *Journal of the American Medical Association* 44 (1905): 1470.

46. J. M. Dodson, "What Shall the Standard Be for Recognition of Medical Colleges and How Shall Such Standard Be Determined?" *Journal of the American Medical Association* 44 (1905): 1474.

47. V. C. Vaughan, "Report of the Committee on Requirements for Admission to Medical Schools," *Journal of the American Medical Association* 44 (1905): 1471–72.

48. Ibid.

49. A. D. Bevan, "Report of the Council on Medical Education to the House of Delegates, July 10, 1905," *Journal of the American Medical Association* 45 (1905): 270.

50. M. A. Fishbein, *History of the American Medical Association,* 895.

51. S. Lewis, *Arrowsmith* (New York: Penguin Group, 1998), 7.

Chapter 3 · *A National Standard for Premedical Education*

1. J. L. Wilson, "Stanford University School of Medicine and the Predecessor Schools: An Historical Perspective," available at http://elane.stanford.edu/wilson.

2. Ibid., chap. 27.

3. Ibid., chap. 28.

4. Statutes of California, 1901, Chapter LI, pp. 56–64.

5. Ibid., 58.

6. Association of American Medical Colleges, "Regarding the requirements for admission to be maintained by colleges belonging to this Association," *Journal of the American Medical Association* 37 (1901): 757.

7. Ibid.

8. Wilson, "Stanford University School of Medicine," chap. 28.

9. C. J. Blake, letter to President Jordan, Leland Stanford Junior University, September 17, 1902, Department of Special Collections, Stanford University Libraries.

10. Wilson, "Stanford University School of Medicine," chap. 29.

11. G. Crothers, Report to the Trustees, November 1, 1906, Department of Special Collections, Stanford University Libraries.

12. The Leland Stanford Junior University, *First Annual Register,* 1891–92, 75.

13. The Leland Stanford Junior University, *Fourth Annual Register,* 1893/94, 103.

14. D. S. Jordan, Letter to Stanford University Trustees, September 14, 1907, Department of Special Collections, Stanford University Libraries.

15. D. S. Jordan, "Fifth Annual Report of the President of the University for the Year Ending July 31, 1908," 19; Leland Stanford Junior University, *Eighteenth Annual Register,* 1908/9, 167.

16. A. D. Bevan, "Cooperation in Medical Education and Medical Service—Functions of the Medical Profession, of the University and of the Public," *Journal of the American Medical Association* 90 (1928): 1174.

17. Ibid., 1175.

18. Ibid.

19. Ibid.

20. K. M. Ludmerer, *Learning to Heal: The Development of American Medical Education* (Baltimore: Johns Hopkins University Press, 1996), 170.

21. Council on Medical Education, Minutes of the meeting of December 1908, as quoted in M. Fishbein, *History of the American Medical Association,* 898.

22. A. Flexner, *I Remember: The Autobiography of Abraham Flexner* (New York: Simon and Schuster, 1940), 60.

23. Ibid., 97.

24. Ludmerer, *Learning to Heal,* 172.

25. Flexner, *I Remember,* 110.

26. Ibid., 114.

27. A. Flexner, from "Reminiscences of Dr. Welch," 1934, as quoted in Ludmerer, *Learning to Heal,* 172.

28. Flexner, *I Remember,* 115.

29. T. N. Bonner, *Iconoclast: Abraham Flexner and a Life of Learning* (Baltimore: Johns Hopkins University Press, 2002), 77.

30. Flexner, *I Remember,* 121.

31. A. Flexner, *Medical Education in the United States and Canada* (New York: Carnegie Foundation for the Advancement of Teaching, 1910), 23.

32. Flexner, *I Remember,* 52.

33. Flexner, *Medical Education in the United States,* 24–26.

34. Ludmerer, *Learning to Heal,* 184.

35. Fishbein, *History of the American Medical Association,* 898.

36. A. M. Bevan, "Medicine a Function of the State," *Journal of the American Medical Association* 42 (1914): 821.

37. V. C. Vaughan, "Remarks Made to the Tenth Annual Conference of the Council on Medical Education," *American Medical Association Bulletin* 9 (1914): 294.

38. A. L. Lowell, "The Danger to the Maintenance of High Standards of Excessive Formalism," *Journal of the American Medical Association* 42 (1914): 824.

39. Ibid., 824.

40. Ibid.

41. Ibid., 825.

42. Association of American Medical Colleges, "Minimum Entrance Requirements," *Bulletin of the Association of American Medical Colleges* 1(1) (1926): 22–24.

43. H. Cabot, "The Premedical Course," *Bulletin of the Association of American Medical Colleges* 1(1) (1926): 2.

44. Ibid., 1–2.

45. S. P. Capen, "Premedical Education," *Bulletin of the Association of American Medical Colleges* 1(1) (1926): 5.

46. Ibid., 8.

47. F. B. Barker, "Determining the Fitness of the Premedical Student," *Bulletin of the Association of American Medical Colleges* 2(1) (1927): 18–19.

48. W. C. Rappleye, "Medical Education," *Journal of Higher Education* 1 (1930): 156.

49. Association of American Medical Colleges, *Final Report of the Commission on Medical Education* (New York: Office of the Director of the Study, 1932). Hereafter, references to this report are in parenthetical page numbers in the text.

50. H. H. Plough, "Medical Schools and Pre-medical Training," A talk delivered to the Pre-medical Club at Amherst College, November 19, 1936, Amherst College Library, Archives and Special Collections.

51. F. J. Mullen, "Selection of Medical Students," *Journal of the Association of American Medical Colleges* 23 (1948): 164.

52. D. B. Tressider, "The Aims and Purpose of Medical Education," *Journal of the Association of American Medical Colleges* 23 (1948): 2–17.

53. A. E. Severinghaus, H. J. Carmen, and W. E. Cadbury, *Preparation for Medical Education in the Liberal Arts Colleges: The Report of the Subcommittee on Preprofessional Education of the Survey of Medical Education* (New York: McGraw-Hill, 1953), 1.

54. Ibid., 9.

55. Ibid., 11.

56. Ibid.

57. Ibid., 99.

58. D. C. Gilman, Address given on Commemoration Day, Johns Hopkins University, February 22, 1893, Alan Mason Chesney Archives, Johns Hopkins Medical Institutions.

59. Severinghaus, Carmen, and Cadbury, *Preparation for Medical Education,* 1953, 14.

60. Ibid., 72.

61. D. H. Funkenstein, "Some Myths about Medical School Admissions," *Journal of Medical Education* 30 (1955): 81.

62. H. H. Gee and J. T. Cowles, *The Appraisal of Applicants to Medical Schools: Report of the Fourth Teaching Institute of the Association of American Medical Colleges, November 7–10, 1956* (Evanston, IL: Association of American Medical Colleges, 1957).

63. T. R. McConnell, "Reflections on Medical Education and Some of the Problems of Selection," in Gee and Cowles, *Appraisal of Applicants to Medical Schools,* 16–21.

64. Funkenstein, "Some Myths about Medical School Admissions," 88.

65. G. E. Miller, ed., *Teaching and Learning in Medical School* (Cambridge: Harvard University Press, 1961), 4, 10.

66. L. Thomas, "How to Fix the Premedical Curriculum," *New England Journal of Medicine* 298 (1978): 1180.

67. G. H. Breiger, "The Plight of Premedical Education: Myths and Misperceptions—Part I: The Premedical Syndrome," *Academic Medicine* 74 (1999): 901–4; Breiger, "The Plight of Premedical Education: Myths and Misperceptions—Part II: Science 'versus' the Liberal Arts," *Academic Medicine* 74 (1999): 1217–21.

68. R. L. Dickman, R. E. Sarnacki, F. T. Schimpfhauser, and L. A. Katz, "Medical Students from Natural Science and Non-science Undergraduate Backgrounds: Similar Academic Performance and Residency Selection," *JAMA* 243 (1980): 2506–9.

69. C. Zeleznik, M. Hojat M, and J. Veloski, "Baccalaureate Preparation for Medical School: Does Type of Degree Make a Difference?" *Journal of Medical Education* 58 (1983): 26–33.

70. B. Doblin and S. Korenman, "The Role of Natural Sciences in the Premedical Curriculum," *Academic Medicine* 67 (1992): 539–41.

71. E. D. Pellegrino, "Pruning an Old Root: Premedical Science and Medical School," *JAMA* 243 (1980): 2518–19.

72. Dickman, Sarnacki, Schimpfhauser, and Katz, "Medical Students," 2509.

73. Pellegrino, "Pruning an Old Root," 2518.

74. P. J. Imperato, "The Need for Premedical Curricular Reform," *Academic Medicine* 72 (1997): 734.

75. J. L. Houpt, R. J. Anderson, and C. D. DeAngelis, "In Reply," *Academic Medicine* 72 (1997): 734.

76. E. J. Emanuel, "Changing Premed Requirements," *JAMA* 296 (2006): 1129.

Chapter 4 • Premedical Education and the Prediction of Professional Performance

1. F. C. Zapffe, "Study of Applicants for Admission to the 1935 Freshman Class in Seventy-nine Medical Schools," *Journal of the Association of American Medical Colleges* 11 (1936): 185–200.

2. B. D. Myers, "Report of Applications for Matriculation in Schools of Medicine for 1927–1928," *Bulletin of the Association of American Medical Colleges* 3 (1928): 193–99.

3. J. Wyckoff, "Relation of Collegiate Scholarship to Medical Student Scholarship," *Bulletin of the Association of American Medical Colleges* 2 (1927): 1.

4. Ibid.

5. Ibid., 12.

6. F. T. van Beuren Jr., "Correlation of Grades in Medical and Premedical Work with Personality," *Journal of the Association of American Medical Colleges* 4 (1929): 199.

7. D. A. Robertson, "Educational Relations of the Professions," *Journal of the American Medical Association* 92 (1929): 1403.

8. A. L. Lowell, "The Danger to the Maintenance of High Standards of Excessive Formalism," *Journal of the American Medical Association* 42 (1914): 824.

9. A. L. Lowell, "College Studies and Professional Training," *Educational Review* 42 (1911): 217–33.

10. Ibid., 224.

11. Ibid., 227.

12. Myers, "Report of Applications," 198.

13. M. A. May, "Predicting Academic Success," *Journal of Educational Psychology* 14 (1923): 439.

14. N. Leman, *The Big Test: The Secret History of the American Meritocracy* (New York: Farrar, Strauss, and Giroux, 1999), 18.

15. Ibid., 24.

16. M. V. Cobb and R. M. Yerkes, "Intellectual and Educational Status of the Medical Profession as Represented in the United States Army," *Bulletin of the National Research Council* 1 (1921): (Part 8 Number 8) 458–532.

17. Robertson, "Educational Relations of the Professions."

18. Ibid., 1404.

19. Ibid., 1406.

20. F. A. Moss, "Scholastic Aptitude Test for Medical Students," *Journal of the Association of American Medical Colleges* 5 (1930): 90–110.

21. Ibid., 96.

22. Ibid., 110.

23. A. M. Chesney, W. Hale, E. S. Thorpe, and C. E. Palmer, "Evaluation of the Medical Aptitude Test," *Journal of the Association of American Medical Colleges* 11 (1936): 17.

24. E. L. Thorndike, Letter to Alan M. Chesney, October 7, 1935, responding to Chesney et al., "Evaluation of the MAT," 26.

25. F. A. Moss, "Report of the Committee on Aptitude Tests for Medical School," *Journal of the Association of American Medical Colleges* 13 (1938): 177–89.

26. F. A. Moss, "Report of the Committee on Aptitude Tests for Medical School," *Journal of the Association of American Medical Colleges* 15 (1940): 249–55.

27. C. F. Cramer, "A Study of the Selective Admission of Students in the Medical Schools of the University of Chicago," *Journal of the Association of American Medical Colleges* 8 (1933): 349.

28. I. L. Kandel, *Professional Aptitude Tests in Medicine, Law, and Engineering* (New York: Teachers College, Columbia University, 1940), viii.

29. Moss, "Report of the Committee on Aptitude Tests" (1940), 255.

30. R. B. Ralph and C. W. Taylor, "A Comparative Evaluation of the Professional Aptitude Test and the General Aptitude Test Battery," *Journal of the Association of American Medical Colleges* 25 (1948): 33.

31. Ibid., 40.

32. J. K. Hill, "Assessment of Intellectual Promise for Medical School," *Journal of Medical Education* 34 (1959): 959–64.

33. E. Gottheil and C. M. Michael, "Predictor Variables Employed in Research on the Selection of Medical Students," *Journal of Medical Education* 32 (1957): 131, 135.

34. H. H. Gee and J. T. Cowles, eds., *The Appraisal of Applicants to Medical School: Report of the Fourth Teaching Institute of the Association of American Medical Colleges, November 7–10, 1956* (Evanston, IL: Association of American Medical Colleges, 1957), 9.

35. R. J. Glaser, "Appraising Intellectual Characteristics," in Gee and Cowles, *Appraisal of Applicants to Medical School,* 31–43.

36. Ibid., 34.

37. D. Wolfe, "Medicine's Share in America's Student Resources," in Gee and Cowles, *Appraisal of Applicants Medical School,* 14.

38. R. F. Arragon, "The Place of the College in Selection and Preparation for Medicine," in Gee and Cowles, *Appraisal of Applicants to Medical School,* 165.

39. Glaser, "Appraising Intellectual Characteristics," 41.

40. J. L. Caughey, "Introduction to the Methods and Goals of Medical Student Selection," in Gee and Cowles, *Appraisal of Applicants to Medical School,* 175–76.

41. A. E. Schwartzman, R. C. A. Hunter, and J. G. Lohrenz, "Factors Related to Medical School Achievement," *Journal of Medical Education* 37 (1962): 749–59.

42. D. H. Funkenstein, "Failure to Graduate from Medical School," *Journal of Medical Education* 37 (1962): 588–603.

43. H. G. Gough and W. B. Hall, "An Attempt to Predict Graduation from Medical School," *Journal of Medical Education* 50 (1975): 940–50.

44. M. Korman, R. L. Stubblefield, and L. W. Martin, "Faculty and Student Perceptions of Medical Roles," *Journal of Medical Education* 39 (1964): 197–202; Korman, Stubblefield, and Martin, "Patterns of Success in Medical School and Their Correlates," *Journal of Medical Education* 43 (1968): 405–11; Korman and Stubblefield, "Medical School Evaluation and Intern Performance," *Journal of Medical Education* 46 (1971): 670–73.

45. J. M. Richards Jr., C. W. Taylor, and P. B. Price, "The Prediction of Medical Intern Performance," *Journal of Applied Psychology* 46 (1962): 142.

46. M. A. Howell and J. W. Vincent, "The Medical College Admission Test as Related to Achievement Tests in Medicine and to Supervisory Evaluations of Clinical Physicians," *Journal of Medical Education* 42 (1967): 1037–44.

47. V. Johnson, R. D. Miller, and R. P. Gage, "Correlation between Performance in Medical School and Residency Training," *Journal of Medical Education* 38 (1963): 591–95.

48. P. B. Price, C. W. Taylor, J. M. Richards, and T. L. Jacobsen, "Measurement of Physician Performance," *Journal of Medical Education* 39 (1964): 208.

49. Ibid., 211.

50. H. G. Gough, W. B. Hall, and R. E. Harris, "Admissions Procedures as Forecasters of Performance in Medical Training," *Journal of Medical Education* 38 (1963): 983–98; Gough, Hall, and Harris, "Evaluation of Performance in Medical Training," *Journal of Medical Education* 39 (1964): 679–92; P. B. Price et al., "Measurement and Predictors of Physician Performance: Two Decades of Intermittently Sustained Research," U.S. Department of Health, Education and Welfare, PB-224 543, 1971; J. R. Wingard and J. W. Williamson, "Grades as Predictors of Physicians' Career Performance: An Evaluation Literature Review," *Journal of Medical Education* 48 (1973): 311–22.

51. Gough, Hall, and Harris, "Admissions Procedures" (1963), 994.

52. Wingard and Williamson, "Grades as Predictors" (1973), 311.

53. M. W. Herman and J. J. Veloski, "Premedical Training, Personal Characteristics and Performance in Medical School," *Medical Education* 15 (1981): 363–67; Herman, Veloski, M. Hojat, "Validity and Importance of Low Ratings Given Medical Graduates in Noncognitive Areas," *Journal of Medical Education* 58 (1983): 837–43.

54. R. A. DeVaul et al., "Medical School Performance of Initially Rejected Students," *JAMA* 257 (1987): 47.

55. K. J. Mitchell, "Traditional Predictors of Performance in Medical School," *Academic Medicine* 65 (1990): 149–58.

56. K. Glaser, M. Hojat, J. J. Veloski, R. S. Blacklow, and C. E. Goepp, "Science, Verbal, Or Quantitative Skills: Which Is the Most Important Predictor of Physician Competence?" *Educational and Psychological Measurement* 52 (1992): 395–406.

57. Ibid., 404.

58. L. A. Loftus, L. Arnold, T. L. Willoughby, A. Connolly, "First-year Residents' Performance Compared with Their Medical School Class Rank as Determined by Three Ranking Systems," *Academic Medicine* 67 (1992): 319–23.

59. N. D. Anderson, "The Mismeasure of Medical Education," *Academic Medicine* 65 (1990): 159–60; W. C. McGaghie, "Assessing Readiness for Medical Education—Evolution of the Medical College Admissions Test," *JAMA* 288 (2002): 1085–90.

60. Association of American Medical Colleges, "Preparing for the MCAT Exam," available at www.aamc.org/students/mcat/preparing/start.htm.

61. D. B. Swanson, S. M. Case, J. Koenig, and C. D. Killian, "Preliminary Study of the Old and New Medical College Admissions Tests for Predicting Performance on USMLE Step I," *Academic Medicine* 71 (1996): S25–S27.

62. A. Wiley and J. A. Koenig, "The Validity of the Medical College Admissions Tests for Predicting Performance in the First Two Years of Medical School," *Academic Medicine* 71 (1996): S83–S85.

63. E. R. Julian, "Validity of the Medical College Admissions Tests for Predicting Medical School Performance," *Academic Medicine* 80 (2005): 910–17.

64. J. J. Veloski, C. A. Callahan, G. Xu, M. Hojat, and D. B. Nash, "Prediction of Students' Performances on Licensing Examinations Using Age, Race, Sex, Undergraduate GPAs, and MCAT Scores," *Academic Medicine* 75 (2000): S28–S30.

65. T. Donnon, E. O. Paolucci, and C. Violato, "The Predictive Validity of the MCAT for Medical School Performance and Medical Board Licensing Examinations: A Meta-analysis of the Published Research, *Academic Medicine* 82 (2007): 100–106.

66. M. Hojat, J. B. Erdmann, J. J. Veloski et al., "A Validity Study of the Writing Sample Section of the Medical College Admission Test, *Academic Medicine* 75 (2000): S25–S27.

67. Ibid., S27.

68. M. A. Papadakis, "The Step 2 Clinical-Skills Examination," *New England Journal of Medicine* 350 (2004): 1703–5.

69. N. V. Vu, H. S. Barrows, M. L. Marcy et al., "Six Years of Comprehensive, Clinical, Performance-Based Assessment Using Standardized Patients at the Southern Illinois University School of Medicine," *Academic Medicine* 67 (1992): 48.

70. J. A. Colliver, M. H. Swartz, R. S. Robbs, and D. S. Cohen, "Relationship between Clinical Competence and Interpersonal and Communication Skills in Standardized Patient Assessment," *Academic Medicine* 74 (1999): 271–74.

71. W. T. Basco, G. E. Gilbert, A. W. Chessman, and A. V. Blue, "The Ability of a Medical School Admission Process to Predict Clinical Performance and Patients' Satisfaction," *Academic Medicine* 75 (2000): 743–47.

72. R. A. Edelstein, H. M. Reid, R. Usatine, and M. S. Wilkes, "A Comparative Study of Measures to Evaluate Medical Students' Performance," *Academic Medicine* 75 (2000): 825–33.

73. R. K. Reznick, D. Blackmore, W. D. Dauphinée, A. I. Rothman, and S. Smee, "Large-Scale High-Stakes Testing with an OSCE: Report from the Medical Council of Canada," *Academic Medicine* 71 (1996): S19–S21.

74. C. Violato and T. Donnon, "Does the Medical College Admission Test Predict Clinical Reasoning Skills? A Longitudinal Study Employing the Medical Council of Canada Clinical Reasoning Examination," *Academic Medicine* 80 (2005): S14–S16.

75. R. Tamblyn, M. Abrahamowicz, W. D. Dauphinée et al., "Physician Scores on a National Clinical Skills Examination as Predictors of Complaints to Medical Regulatory Authorities," *JAMA* 298 (2007): 993–1001.

76. Ibid., 997.

77. G. Makoul and R. H. Curry, "The Value of Assessing and Addressing Communication Skills," *JAMA* 298 (2007): 1057–59.

78. D. G. Johnson and E. B. Hutchins, "Doctor or Dropout? A Study of Medical School Attrition," special edition, *Journal of Medical Education* 41 (1966): 1099–1204.

79. Association of American Medical Colleges, "Applicants, First-Time Applicants, Acceptees, and Matriculants to U.S. Medical Schools by Sex, 1996–2007, and Total Graduates from U.S. Medical Schools by Sex, 2002–2007," available at www.aamc.org/data/facts/start.htm.

Chapter 5 · Noncognitive Factors That Predict Professional Performance

1. E. S. Thorpe, "Relative Value of Cultural Courses in Premedical Training," *Journal of the Association of American Medical Colleges* 6 (1931): 80.

2. E. P. Lyon, "Cultural Value of the Medical Curriculum," *Journal of the Association of American Medical Colleges* 6 (1931): 85.

3. J. Wyckoff, "Relation of Collegiate Scholarship to Medical Student Scholarship," *Bulletin of the Association of American Medical Colleges* 2 (1927): 1.

4. R. J. Glaser, "Appraising Intellectual Characteristics," chapter 3 in Gee and Cowles, eds., *Appraisal of Applicants to Medical School* (Evanston, IL: Association of American Medical Colleges, 1957).

5. J. J. Ceithaml, "Appraising Nonintellectual Characteristics," chapter 4 in Gee and Cowles, eds. *Appraisal of Applicants to Medical School.*

6. Ibid., 56.

7. Gee and Cowles, *Appraisal of Applicants to Medical School,* 60.

8. J. S. Handler, "The Selection of Medical Students via the Psychiatric Interview," in Gee and Cowles, *Appraisal of Applicants to Medical School,* 67–72.

9. Ibid., 68.

10. C. F. Schumacher, "Personal Characteristics of Students Choosing Different Types of Medical Careers," *Journal of Medical Education* 39 (1964): 278–88.

11. E. B. Hutchins, "The AAMC Longitudinal Study: Implications for Medical Education," *Journal of Medical Education* 39 (1964): 265–77.

12. J. L. Caughey, "Nonintellectual Components of Medical Education," *Journal of Medical Education* 42 (1967): 619.

13. J. Parlow and A. I. Rothman, "Personality Traits of First-year Medical Students: Trends over a Six-year Period, 1967–1972," *British Journal of Medical Education* 8 (1974): 8–12.

14. J. V. Haley and M. J. Lerner, "The Characteristics and Performance of Medical Students During Clinical Training," *Journal of Medical Education* 47 (1972): 451.

15. Ibid., 452.

16. E. V. Turner, M. M. Helper, S. D. Kriska, "Predictors of Clinical Performance," *Journal of Medical Education* 49 (1974): 338–42.

17. H. G. Gough, "Some Predictive Implications of Premedical Scientific Competence and Preferences," *Journal of Medical Education* 53 (1978): 291.

18. H. G. Gough and W. B. Hall, "An Attempt to Predict Graduation from Medical School," *Journal of Medical Education* 50 (1975): 940–50.

19. Gough, "Some Predictive Implications," 298.

20. G. D. Miller, D. Frank, R. D. Franks, and C. J. Getto, "Noncognitive Criteria for Assessing Students in North American Medical Schools," *Academic Medicine* 64 (1989): 42–45.

21. G. I. Feletti, R. W. Sanson-Fisher, M. Vidler, and the Admissions Committee of the Faculty of Medicine, University of Newcastle, New South Wales, "Evaluating a New Approach to Selecting Medical Students," *Medical Education* 19 (1985): 276–84.

22. C. K. Aldrich, "Psychiatric Interviews and Psychological Tests as Predictors of Medical Students' Success," *Journal of Medical Education* 62 (1987): 658–64.

23. M. Hojat, M. Robeson, I. Damjanov et al., "Students' Psychological Characteristics as Predictors of Academic Performance in Medical School," *Academic Medicine* 68 (1993): 636.

24. M. Hojat, K. M. Glaser, and J. J. Veloski, "Associations between Selected Psychosocial Attributes and Rating of Physician Competence," *Academic Medicine* 71 (1996): S104, S105.

25. W. C. McGaghie, "Perspectives on Medical School Admission" and "Qualitative Variables in Medical School Admission," *Academic Medicine* 65 (1990): 136–39, 145–49.

26. Ibid., 145.

27. H. Shen and A. L. Comrey, "Predicting Medical Students' Academic Performances by Their Cognitive Abilities and Personality Characteristics," *Academic Medicine* 72 (1997): 781–86.

28. L. D. Cariaga-Lo, C. E. Enarson, S. J. Crandall, D. J. Zaccaro, and B. F. Richards, "Cognitive and Noncognitive Predictors of Academic Difficulty and Attrition," *Academic Medicine* 72 (1997): S69–S71.

29. R. M. Carrothers, S. W. Gregory, and T. J. Gallagher, "Measuring Emotional Intelligence of Medical School Applicants," *Academic Medicine* 75 (2000): 460.

30. R. S. Manuel, N. J. Borges, and H. A. Gerzina, "Personality and Clinical Skills: Any Correlation?" *Academic Medicine* 80 (2005): S30–S33.

31. Medical School Objectives Writing Group, "Learning Objectives for Medical Student Education—Guidelines for Medical Schools: Report I of the Medical School Objectives Project," *Academic Medicine* 74 (1999): 13–18.

32. W. C. McGaghie, "Assessing Readiness for Medical Education—Evolution of the Medical College Admissions Test," *JAMA* 288 (2002): 1085–90.

33. M. A. Albanese, M. H. Snow, S. E. Skochelak, K. N. Huggett, and P. M. Farrell, "Assessing Personal Qualities in Medical School Admissions," *Academic Medicine* 78 (2003): 313–21.

34. E. Ferguson, D. James, and L. Madeley, "Factors Associated with Success in Medical School: Systematic Review of the Literature," *BMJ* 324 (2002): 952–57.

35. Ceithaml, "Appraising Nonintellectual Characteristics," 44.

36. Ibid., 53.

37. Ibid., 54.

38. J. Zubin, "A Brief Survey of the Interview," in Gee and Cowles, eds., *Appraisal of Applicants to Medical School,* 63.

39. E. L. Kelley, "A Critique of the Interview," in Gee and Cowles, eds., *Appraisal of Applicants to Medical School,* 78–84.

40. Ibid., 84.

41. J. C. Edwards, E. K. Johnson, and J. B. Molidor, "The Interview in the Admission Process," *Academic Medicine* 65 (1990): 167–77.

42. T. C. Taylor, "The Interview: One More Life," *Academic Medicine* 65 (1990): 178.

43. P. H. Harasym, W. Woloschuk, H. Mandin, and R. Brundin-Mather, "Reliability and Validity of Interviewers' Judgments of Medical School Candidates," *Academic Medicine* 71 (1996): S40–S42.

44. C. L. Elam and M. M. S. Johnson, "An Analysis of Admission Committee Voting Patterns," *Academic Medicine* 71 (1996): S72–S75.

45. J. C. Georgesen, J. F. Wilson, C. L. Elam, and K. S. Stahlman, "Academic and Noncognitive Factors Affecting Placement of Medical School Applicants on an Alternate List," *Academic Medicine* 74 (1999): S65–S67.

46. L. E. Patrick, E. M. Altmaier, S. Kuperman, and K. Ugolini, "A Structured Interview for Medical School Admission, Phase 1: Initial Procedures and Results," *Academic Medicine* 76 (2001): 66–71.

47. S. Muller, Introduction to "Physicians for the Twenty-First Century—Report of the Project Panel on the General Professional Education of the Physician and College Preparation for Medicine, Association of American Medical Colleges," *Journal of Medical Education* 59 (11 Part 2) (1984): 1.

48. M. H. Davis, "Measuring Individual Differences in Empathy: Evidence for a Multidimensional Approach," *Journal of Personality and Social Psychology* 44 (1983): 113–26.

49. D. J. Kupfer, F. L. Drew, E. K. Curtis, and D. N. Rubinstein, "Personality Style and Empathy in Medical Students," *Journal of Medical Education* 53 (1978): 507–9.

50. W. T. Branch Jr., R. J. Pels, and J. P. Hafler, "Medical Students' Empathetic Understanding of Their Patients," *Academic Medicine* 73 (1998): 360.

51. E. R. Marcus, "Empathy, Humanism, and the Professionalization Process of Medical Education," *Academic Medicine* 74 (1999): 1211–15.

52. R. A. Diseker and R. Michielutte, "An Analysis of Empathy in Medical Students Before and Following Clinical Experience," *Journal of Medical Education* 56 (1981): 1004–10.

53. C. P. West, J. L. Huntington, M. M. Huschka et al., "A Prospective Study of the Relationship between Medical Knowledge and Professionalism among Internal Medicine Residents," *Academic Medicine* 82 (2007): 587–92.

54. P. J. Tutton, "Psychometric Test Results Associated with High Achievement in Basic Science Components of a Medical Curriculum," *Academic Medicine* 71 (1996): 181–86.

55. Ibid., 185.

56. D. Lubinski, "Introduction to the Special Section on Cognitive Abilities: 100 Years After Spearman's (1904) '"General Intelligence," Objectively Determined and Measured,'" *Journal of Personality and Social Psychology* 86, no. 1 (2004): 96–111.

57. Ibid., 103.

58. H. A. Witkin, C. A. Moore, P. K. Oltman et al., "Role of Field-Dependent and Field-Independent Cognitive Styles in Academic Evolution: A Longitudinal Study," *Journal of Educational Psychology* 69 (1977): 197–211.

59. J. A. Richardson and T. E. Turner, "Field Dependence Revisited: Intelligence," *Educational Psychology* 20 (2000): 255–70.

60. H. A. Witkin and D. R. Goodenough, "Field Dependence and Interpersonal Behavior," *Psychological Bulletin* 84 (1977): 661.

61. Tutton, "Psychometric Test Results," 185.

62. M. Hojat, J. S. Gonnella, S. Mangione et al., "Empathy in Medical Students as Related to Academic Performance, Clinical Competence, and Gender," *Medical Education* 36 (2002): 522–27.

63. T. D. Stratton, C. L. Elam, A. E. Murphy-Spencer, and S. L. Quinlivan, "Emotional Intelligence and Clinical Skills: Preliminary Results from a Comprehensive Clinical Performance Examination," *Academic Medicine* 80 (2005): S35.

64. A. D. Poole and R. W. Sanson-Fisher, "Long-Term Effects of Empathy Training on the Interview Skills of Medical Students," *Patient Counseling and Health Education* 2 (3) (1980): 125–27.

65. C. E. Rees and L. V. Knight, "The Trouble with Assessing Students' Professionalism: Theoretical Insights from Sociocognitive Psychology," *Academic Medicine* 82 (2007): 46–50.

66. J. Benbassat and R. Baumal R., "What Is Empathy, and How Can It Be Promoted during Clinical Clerkships?" *Academic Medicine* 79 (2004): 834.

67. B. W. Newton, L. Barber, J. Clardy, E. Cleveland, and P. O'Sullivan, "Is There Hardening of the Heart During Medical School?" *Academic Medicine* 83 (2008): 244–49.

68. H. Spiro, "What Is Empathy and Can It Be Taught?" *Annals of Internal Medicine* 116 (1992): 843.

69. G. E. Pence, "Can Compassion Be Taught?" *Journal of Medical Ethics* 9 (1983): 189–90.

70. J. Coulehan and P. C. Williams, "Vanquishing Virtue: The Impact of Medical Education," *Academic Medicine* 76 (2001): 599–601.

71. Kupfer, Drew, Curtis, and Rubinstein, "Personality Style and Empathy," 509.

Chapter 6 · Efforts to Increase the Diversity of the Medical Profession

1. Association of American Medical Colleges, "Diversity in the Physician Workforce: Facts & Figures 2006," available at www.aamc.org/diversity/reading.htm.

2. R. C. Davidson and R. Montoya, "The Distribution of Services to the Underserved: A Comparison of Minority and Majority Medical Graduates in California," *Western Journal of Medicine* 146 (1987): 114–17.

3. Association of American Medical Colleges, "Diversity in the Physician Workforce."

4. *Regents of the University of California v. Bakke,* 438 U.S. 265 (1978).

5. Association of American Medical Colleges, "Diversity in the Physician Workforce."

6. D. A. Evans, P. K. Jones, R. A. Wortman, and E. B. Jackson, "Traditional Criteria as Predictors of Minority Student Success in Medical School," *Journal of Medical Education* 50 (1975): 934–39.

7. Ibid., 938.

8. B. Dawson, C. K. Iwamoto, L. P. Ross et al., "Performance on the National Board of Medical Examiners Part I Examination by Men and Women of Different Race," *JAMA* 272 (1994): 674–79.

9. Ibid., 679.

10. S. N. Keith, R. M. Bell, A. G. Swanson, and A. P. Williams, "Effects of Affirmative Action in Medical Schools: A Study of the Class of 1975," *New England Journal of Medicine* 313 (1985): 1519–25.

11. Ibid., 1524.

12. R. C. Davidson and R. Montoya, "The Distribution of Services to the Underserved: A Comparison of Minority and Majority Medical Graduates in California," *Western Journal of Medicine* 146 (1987): 114–17.

13. R. C. Davidson and J. Fox-Garcia, "Board Certification Rates of Majority and Minority Graduates of Seven California Medical Schools," *Journal of Medical Education* 63 (1988): 656.

14. R. C. Davidson and E. L. Lewis, "Affirmative Action and Other Special Consideration Admissions at the University of California, Davis, School of Medicine," *JAMA* 278 (1997): 1153–58.

15. See K. B. Lynch and M. K. Woode, "The Relationship of Minority Students' MCAT Scores and Grade Point Averages to Their Acceptance into Medical School," *Academic Medicine* 65 (1990): 480–82; L. G. Croen, M. Reichgott, and R. K. Spencer, "A Performance-based Method for Early Identification of Medical Students at Risk of Developing Academic Problems," *Academic Medicine* 66 (1991): 486–88; D. Campos-Outcalt, P. J. Rutala, D. B. Witzke, and J. V. Fulginiti, "Performance of Underrepresented-minority Students at the University of Arizona College of Medicine, 1987–1991," *Academic Medicine* 69 (1994): 577–82.

16. W. E. Sedlacke and D. O. Prieto, "Predicting Minority Students' Success in Medical School," *Academic Medicine* 65 (1990): 161–66.

17. A. Tekian, "A Thematic Review of the Literature on Underrepresented Minorities and Medical Training, 1981–1995: Securing the Foundation of the Bridge to Diversity," *Academic Medicine* 72 (1997): S143.

18. J. A. Koenig, S. G. Sireci, and A. Wiley, "Evaluating the Predictive Validity of MCAT Scores across Diverse Applicant Groups," *Academic Medicine* 73 (1998): 1095–106.

19. S. S. Anderson, "Pipeline Programs: Looking Forward to Promote Diversity," available at www.aamc.org/newsroom/reporter/septo3/pipeline.htm.

20. C. Terrell, "The Health Professions Partnership Initiative and Working Toward Diversity in the Health Care Workforce," *Academic Medicine* 81 (2006): S2.

21. See www.hppi-2020.org/HPPIhome.cfm.

22. M. Slater and E. Iler, "Mount Sinai HPPI," *Academic Medicine* 81 (2006): S41–S43.

23. K. Flores and B. Dominguez, "University of California, San Francisco, Fresno Latino Center for Medical Education and Research Health Professions Pipeline Program," *Academic Medicine* 81 (2006): S36–S40.

24. M. A. Winkleby, "The Stanford Medical Youth Science Program: 18 Years of a Biomedical Program for Low-Income High School Students," *Academic Medicine* 82 (2007): 140.

25. M. Soto-Greene, L. Wright, O. D. Gona, and L. A. Feldman, "Minority Enrichment Programs at the New Jersey Medical School: 26 Years in Review," *Academic Medicine* 74 (1999): 387.

26. M. R. Bediako, B. A. McDermott, M. E. Bleich, and J. A. Colliver, "Ventures in Ed-

ucation: A Pipeline to Medical Education for Minority and Economically Disadvantaged Students," *Academic Medicine* 71 (1996): 190–92.

27. J. D. Carline, D. G. Patterson, L. A. Davis, and D. M. Irby, "Precollege Enrichment Programs Intended to Increase the Representation of Minorities in Medicine," *Academic Medicine* 73 (1998): 297.

28. D. G. Patterson and J. D. Carline, "Promoting Minority Access to Health Careers through Health Profession-Public School Partnerships: A Review of the Literature," *Academic Medicine* 81 (2006): S5–S10.

29. See www.rwjf.org/programareas/resources/product.

30. C. Terrell, "The Health Professions Partnership Initiative and Working Toward Diversity in the Health Care Workforce," *Academic Medicine* 81 (2006): S3.

31. V. B. Thurmond and L. L. Cregler, "Why Students Drop Out of the Pipeline to Health Professions Careers: A Follow-up of Gifted Minority High School Students," *Academic Medicine* 74 (1999): 450.

32. Ibid., 451.

33. U.S. Department of Health and Human Services, Bureau of Health Professions, "Health Careers Opportunity Program," available at http://bhpr.hrsa.gov/diversity/hcop/default.htm.

34. U.S. Department of Health and Human Services, Bureau of Health Professions, "Centers of Excellence," available at http://bhpr.hrsa.gov/diversity/coe/default.htm.

35. Robert Wood Johnson Foundation, The Minority Medical Education Program, described at www.rwjf.org/pr/product.jsp?id=14475.

36. L. Bergeisen and J. C. Cantor, "The Minority Medical Education Program," chapter 3 in *To Improve Health and Health Care 2000: The Robert Wood Johnson Foundation Anthology*, ed. S. L. Isaacs and J. R. Knickman, available at www.rwjf.org/files/publications/books/2000/index.html.

37. J. C. Cantor, L. Bergeisen, and L. C. Baker, "Effect on an Intensive Educational Program for Minority College Students and Recent Graduates on the Probability of Acceptance to Medical School," *JAMA* 280 (1998): 772–76.

38. J. D. Carline, D. G. Patterson, L. A. Davis, "Enrichment Programs for Undergraduate College Students Intended to Increase the Representation of Minorities in Medicine," *Academic Medicine* 73 (1998): 299–312.

39. U.S. Department of Health and Human Services, Health Resources and Services Administration, "FY 2009 Budget Justification, Centers of Excellence," available at www.hrsa .gov/about/budgetjustification09/hpcenter.htm.

40. U.S. Department of Health and Human Services, Health Resources and Services Administration, "FY 2009 Budget Justification, Health Careers Opportunity Program," available at www.hrsa.gov/about/budgetjustification09/hpcareers.htm.

41. Association of American Medical Colleges, Postbaccalaureate Premedical Programs, available at http://services.aamc.org/postbac.

42. Bryn Mawr, The Postbaccalaureate Premedical Program, described at www.brynmawr .edu/postbac/home.shtml.

43. University of California, California Postbaccalaureate Consortium, described at https://meded-postbac.ucsd.edu/index.cfm?curpage=home#consortiuminformation.

44. C. F. Whitten, "Postbaccalaureate Program at Wayne State University School of Medicine: A 30-year Report," *Academic Medicine* 74 (1999): 393–96.

45. Wayne State University School of Medicine, Admissions—Minority and Disadvantaged Applicants, described at www.med.wayne.edu/admissions/applying/selection_process .asp.

46. Whitten, "Postbaccalaureate Program at Wayne State," 395.

47. E. W. Jackson, S. McGlinn, M. Rainey, and H. R. Bardo, "MEDPREP—30 Years of Making a Difference," *Academic Medicine* 78 (2003): 448–53.

48. Southern Illinois University, Medical/Dental Education Preparatory Program, described at www.siumed.edu/medprep/prospective.html.

49. Jackson et al., "MEDPREP—30 Years of Making a Difference," 448.

50. E. W. Jackson and S. McGlinn, "Twenty-year Follow-up on an Enrichment Program for Students Preparing for Health Professions Schools," *Academic Medicine* 69 (1994): 925–27.

51. A. W. Blakely and L. G. Broussard, "Blueprint for Establishing an Effective Postbaccalaureate Medical School Pre-entry Program for Educationally Disadvantaged Students," *Academic Medicine* 78 (2003): 440.

52. K. Grumbach and E. Chen, "Effectiveness of University of California Postbaccalaureate Premedical Programs in Increasing Medical School Matriculation for Minority and Disadvantaged Students," *JAMA* 296 (2006): 1079–85.

53. Ibid., 1079.

54. M. Hojat, R. S. Blacklow, M. Robeson, J. J. Veloski, B. D. Borenstein, "Postbaccalaureate Preparation and Performance in Medical School," *Academic Medicine* 65 (1990): 388–91.

55. B. Giordani et al., "Effectiveness of a Formal Post-Baccalaureate Pre-Medicine Program for Underrepresented Minority Students," *Academic Medicine* 76 (2001): 844–48.

56. Ibid., 848.

57. A. Frohna, "'Watch Me Do It': Three Trajectories Toward Medical School Admission in a Post-Baccalaureate, Premedical Program," *Academic Medicine* 74 (1999): S62–64.

58. Thurmond and Cregler, "Why Students Drop Out of the Pipeline."

Chapter 7 · Nontraditional Programs of Medical Education and Their Success in Training Qualified Physicians

1. Definition of *paradigm* from *Oxford English Dictionary,* online edition.

2. V. C. Vaughan, "Remarks Made to the Tenth Annual Conference of the Council on Medical Education," *American Medical Association Bulletin* 9 (1914): 294.

3. Association of American Medical Colleges, Medical School Admission Requirements, 2008–2009.

4. Vaughan, "Remarks," 294.

5. A. Flexner, *Medical Education in the United States and Canada* (New York: Carnegie Foundation for the Advancement of Teaching, 1910), 24.

6. D. B. Kramer, T. S. Higgins, V. U. Collier et al., Comments on "Changing Premedical Requirements," *JAMA* 297 (2007): 37.

7. Association of American Medical Colleges, *Final Report of the Commission on Medical Education* (New York: Office of the Director of the Study, 1932), 288.

8. The Sophie Davis School of Biomedical Education, described at http://med.cuny.edu.

9. S. A. Roman Jr. and M. L. McGanney, "The Sophie Davis School of Biomedical Education: The First 20 Years of a Unique BS-MD Program," *Academic Medicine* 69 (1994): 224–25.

10. Ibid., 225.

11. S. A. Roman Jr., "Addressing the Urban Pipeline Challenge for the Physician Workforce: The Sophie Davis Model," *Academic Medicine* 79 (2004): 1177.

12. Ibid., 1180.

13. Roman and McGanney, "Sophie Davis School of Biomedical Education."

14. Roman, "Addressing the Urban Pipeline Challenge," 1181.

15. B. M. Drees, L. Arnold, and H. S. Jonas, "The University of Missouri-Kansas City School of Medicine: Thirty-Five Years of Experience with a Nontraditional Approach to Medical Education," *Academic Medicine* 82 (2007): 361–69.

16. A. W. Norman and E. V. Calkins, "Curricular Variations in Combined Baccalaureate-M.D. Programs," *Academic Medicine* 67 (1992): 785–91.

17. Association of American Medical Colleges, Medical School Admission Requirements, 2008–2009.

18. W. A. Thomson, P. G. Ferry, J. E. King, C. Martinez-Wedig, and L. H. Michael, "Increasing Access to Medical Education for Students from Medically Underserved Communities: One Program's Success," *Academic Medicine* 78 (2003): 454–59.

19. K. C. Edelin and A. Ugbolue, "Evaluation of an Early Medical School Selection Program for Underrepresented Minority Students," *Academic Medicine* 76 (2001): 1056–59.

20. S. Muller, Introduction, in "Physicians for the Twenty-First Century: Report of the Project Panel on the General Professional Education of the Physician and College Preparation for Medicine, Association of American Medical Colleges," *Journal of Medical Education* 59 (11 Part 2) (1984): 1–200.

21. Commission on Medical Education, *Final Report,* 267.

22. Muller, Introduction, 2, 8.

23. Mount Sinai School of Medicine, Humanities and Medicine Program, available at www.mountsinai.org/Education/School%20of%20Medicine/Medical%20Education.

24. M. R. Rifkin, K. D. Smith, B. D. Stimmel, A. Stagnaro-Green, and N. G. Kase, "The Mount Sinai Humanities and Medicine Program: An Alternative Pathway to Medical School," *Academic Medicine* 75 (10 supp) (2000): S124–S126.

25. Ibid., S124–S125.

26. McMaster University, "Undergraduate MD Program," available at http://65.39.131.180/ContentPage.aspx?name=MD%20Program%20Home.

27. J. D. Hamilton, "The Selection of Medical Students at McMaster University," *Journal of the Royal College of Physicians London* 6 (1972): 348.

28. McMaster University, "Undergraduate MD Program, Admissions," available at http://65.39.131.180/ContentPage.aspx?name=MD_Program_Admissions.

29. B. M. Ferrier, R. G. McAuley, and R. S. Roberts, "The Selection of Medical Students at McMaster University," *Journal of the Royal College of Physicians London* 12 (1978): 365–78.

30. McMaster University, Michael G. DeGroote School of Medicine, MD Program Administration Office.

31. V. R. Neufeld and H. S. Barrows, "The 'McMaster Philosophy': An Approach to Medical Education," *Journal of Medical Education* 49 (1974): 1049.

32. J. D. Hamilton, "The McMaster Curriculum: A Critique," *British Medical Journal* 1(6019) (1976): 1194.

33. Ibid., 1195.

34. C. A. Woodward and R. G. McAuley, "Can the Academic Background of Medical Graduates Be Detected during Internship?" *Canadian Medical Association Journal* 129 (1983): 567–69.

35. Ibid., 569.

36. M. D. Hanson, K. L. Dore, H. I. Reiter, and K. W. Eva, "Medical School Admissions: Revisiting the Veracity and Independence of Completion of an Autobiographical Screening Tool," *Academic Medicine* 82 (10 Suppl.) (2007): S8–S11.

37. K. W. Eva, J. Rosenfeld, H. I. Reiter, and G. R. Norman, "An Admissions OSCE: The Multiple Mini-interview," *Medical Education* 38 (2004): 314–26.

38. Ibid., 325–26.

39. K. W. Eva, H. I. Reiter, J. Rosenfeld, and G. R. Norman, "The Ability of the Multiple Mini-Interview to Predict Preclerkship Performance in Medical School," *Academic Medicine* 79 (10 Suppl) (2004): S40–S42.

40. H. I. Reiter, K. W. Eva, J. Rosenfeld, and G. R. Norman, "Multiple Mini-interviews Predict Clerkship and Licensing Examination Performance," *Medical Education* 41 (2007): 378–84.

41. K. W. Eva and H. I. Reiter, "Where Judgement Fails: Pitfalls in the Selection Process for Medical Personnel," *Advances in Health Sciences Education* 9 (2004): 168.

Chapter 8 · *Reassessing the Premedical Paradigm*

1. A. E. Severinghaus, H. J. Carmen, and W. E. Cadbury, *Preparation for Medical Education in the Liberal Arts Colleges: The Report of the Subcommittee on Preprofessional Education of the Survey of Medical Education* (New York: McGraw-Hill, 1953), 11.

2. Johns Hopkins University Curricular Bulletin, 1877, as quoted by R. H. Fishbein in "Maryland Medical History," *Maryland Medical Journal* 48 (1999): 229.

3. D. H. Funkenstein, "Some Myths about Medical School Admissions," *Journal of Medical Education* 30 (1955): 81.

4. T. S. Kuhn, *The Structure of Scientific Revolutions,* 2nd ed. (Chicago: University of Chicago Press, 1970), 6.

5. Ibid., 10.

6. Ibid., 4.

7. Ibid., 175.

8. Ibid., 5.

9. Ibid., 19.

10. Association of American Medical Colleges, *Final Report of the Commission on Medical Education* (New York: Office of the Director of the Study, 1932), 267.

11. Ibid., 267.

12. Severinghaus, Carmen, and Cadbury, *Preparation for Medical Education.*

13. S. Muller, "Introduction, Physicians for the Twenty-First Century," *Journal of Medical Education* 59 (11 Part 2) (1984): 2.

14. A. Flexner, *Medical Education in the United States and Canada* (New York: Carnegie Foundation for the Advancement of Teaching, 1910), 24.

15. T. R. McConnell, "Reflections on Medical Education and Some of the Problems of Selection," in Gee and Cowles, *Appraisal of Applicants,* 16.

16. Kuhn, *Structure of Scientific Revolutions,* 23.

17. Ibid., 92.

18. Ibid., 145.

19. J. Wyckoff, "Relation of Collegiate Scholarship to Medical Student Scholarship," *Bulletin of the Association of American Medical Colleges* 2 (1927): 1.

20. J. L. Dienstag, "Relevance and Rigor in Premedical Education," *New England Journal of Medicine* 359 (2008): 221.

21. Ibid., 223–24.

Chapter 9 · *Another Way to Structure Premedical Education*

1. J. L. Dienstag, "Relevance and Rigor in Premedical Education," *New England Journal of Medicine* 359 (2008): 223.

2. Association of American Medical Colleges, Howard Hughes Medical Institute, "Scientific Foundations for Future Physicians," 2009, available at www.aamc.org/scientificfoundations.

3. S. Long, and R. Alpern, "Science for Future Physicians," *Science* 324 (2009): 1241.

4. Mount Sinai School of Medicine. Humanities and Medicine Program, described at www.mountsinai.org/Education/School%20of%20Medicine/Medical%20Education.

5. J. D. Hamilton, "The Selection of Medical Students at McMaster University," *Journal of the Royal College of Physicians London* 6 (1972): 348.

6. L. J. Sax, "Undergraduate Science Majors: Gender Differences in Who Goes to Graduate School," *Review of Higher Education* 24 (2001): 153–72; C. L. Colbeck, A. F. Cabrera, and P. T. Terenzini, "Learning Professional Confidence: Linking Teaching Practices, Students' Self-Perceptions, and Gender," *Review of Higher Education* 24 (2001): 173–91; C. H. Middlecamp and B. Subramaniam, "What Is Feminist Pedagogy? Useful Ideas for Teaching Chemistry," *Journal of Chemical Education* 76 (1999): 520–25; E. Seymour and N. M. Hewitt, *Talking about Leaving: Why Undergraduates Leave the Sciences* (Boulder, CO: Westview Press, 1997); J. Margolis and A. Fisher, *Unlocking the Clubhouse: Women in Computing* (Cambridge: MIT Press, 2002); M. Lorenzo, C. H. Crouch, and E. Mazur, "Reducing the Gender Gap in the Physics Classroom," *American Journal of Physics* 74 (2006): 118–22.

7. SRI International, ChemSense—Visualizing Chemistry, described at www.chemsense .org.

8. E. J. Emanuel, "Changing Premed Requirements and the Medical Curriculum," *JAMA* 296 (2006): 1129.

9. D. B. Kramer, T. S. Higgins, V. U. Collier et al., Comments on "Changing Premedical Requirements," *JAMA* 297 (2007): 37–38.